Frozen Section Library

**Series Editor
Philip T. Cagle, MD
Houston, Texas, USA**

For further volumes, go to
http://www.springer.com/series/7869

Frozen Section Library: Head and Neck

Qihui "Jim" Zhai, MD, FCAP

*Department of Pathology & Laboratory Medicine,
University of Cincinnati, Cincinnati, OH, USA*

Including Chapter 6 co-authored by:

Ady Kendler, MD, PhD

University of Cincinnati Medical School, Cincinnati, OH

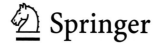 Springer

Qihui "Jim" Zhai
Department of Pathology and Laboratory Medicine
University of Cincinnati
OH, USA
Qihui.Zhai@uc.edu

ISSN 1868-4157   e-ISSN 1868-4165
ISBN 978-0-387-95987-0   e-ISBN 978-0-387-95988-7
DOI 10.1007/978-0-387-95988-7
Springer New York Dordrecht Heidelberg London

Library of Congress Control Number: 2010937990

Springer is part of Springer Science+Business Media (www.springer.com)

To my wife Jenny and daughter Jasmine

Series Preface

For over 100 years, the frozen section has been utilized as a tool for the rapid diagnosis of specimens while a patient is undergoing surgery, usually under general anesthesia, as a basis for making immediate treatment decisions. Frozen section diagnosis is often a challenge for the pathologist who must render a diagnosis that has crucial import for the patient in a minimal amount of time. In addition to the need for rapid recall of differential diagnoses, there are many pitfalls and artifacts that add to the risk of frozen section diagnosis that are not present with permanent sections of fully processed tissues that can be examined in a more leisurely fashion. Despite the century-long utilization of frozen sections, most standard pathology textbooks, both general and subspecialty, largely ignore the topic of frozen sections. Few textbooks have ever focused exclusively on frozen section diagnosis and those textbooks that have done so are now out-of-date and have limited illustrations.

The Frozen Section Library Series is meant to provide convenient, user-friendly handbooks for each organ system to expedite use in the rushed frozen section situation. These books are small and lightweight, copiously color illustrated with images of actual frozen sections, highlighting pitfalls, artifacts, and differential diagnosis. The advantages of a series of organ-specific handbooks, in addition to the ease-of-use and manageable size, are that (1) a series allows more comprehensive coverage of more diagnoses, both common and rare, than a single volume that tries to highlight a limited number of diagnoses for each organ and (2) a series allows more detailed insight by permitting experienced authorities to emphasize the peculiarities of frozen section for each organ system.

As a handbook for practicing pathologists, these books will be indispensable aids to diagnosis and avoiding dangers in one of the most challenging situations that pathologists encounter. Rapid consideration of differential diagnoses and how to avoid traps caused by frozen section artifacts are emphasized in these handbooks. A series of concise, easy-to-use, well-illustrated handbooks alleviates the often frustrating and time-consuming, sometimes futile, process of searching through bulky textbooks that are unlikely to illustrate or discuss pathologic diagnoses from the perspective of frozen sections in the first place. Tables and charts will provide guidance for differential diagnosis of various histologic patterns. Touch preparations, which are used for some organs such as central nervous system or thyroid more often than others, are appropriately emphasized and illustrated according to the need for each specific organ.

This series is meant to benefit practicing surgical pathologists, both community and academic, and to pathology residents and fellows; and also to provide valuable perspectives to surgeons, surgery residents, and fellows who must rely on frozen section diagnosis by their pathologists. Most of all, we hope that this series contributes to the improved care of patients who rely on the frozen section to help guide their treatment.

Houston, TX   Philip T. Cagle, MD
                                                      Series Editor

Preface

Frozen section diagnosis is a critical component of most surgical pathologists' daily practice. Reaching an accurate diagnosis is sometimes stressful considering the time limitations, frozen section artifacts, and the immediate resulting surgical impact. Diseases of the head and neck can be difficult to diagnose because the anatomy is complex and the histology is of a wide spectrum. The origins of these diseases can be epithelial, mesenchymal, melanocytic, and lymphoid, or sometimes a combination. Well-organized chapters or dedicated books that address "pearls" and "pitfalls" in frozen section diagnoses specific to head and neck lesions are rare.

This book as a volume of the Frozen Section Library Series will concentrate on the practical issues commonly encountered in head and neck frozen sections. The contents are a result of both indirect experience from published literature and personal experience. Input from head and neck surgeons has also been incorporated.

The book contains six chapters, beginning with general principles, followed by the diseases from various organs/systems including "Nasal Cavity and Paranasal Sinuses," "Salivary Glands," "Oral Cavity, Pharynx, and Larynx," and "Neck." An additional chapter addressing "Head and Neck Presentations of Intracranial Lesions" is included and dedicated to emphasize the existence of such scenarios.

Each chapter will use a similar format, discussing the importance of communications with the surgeon, understanding the commonly encountered clinical scenarios and indications, suggesting how to handle the specimen appropriately, and highlighting diagnostic pitfalls and pearls. Pathologists should be aware that in the best interest of patient care, deferring to permanent is a valid option for difficult cases in order to avoid an irreversible overtreatment. In some scenarios, a frozen section diagnosis should not be attempted.

I sincerely hope that this book will fill a niche in head and neck pathology, and provide practical, succinct, and yet comprehensive guidelines for the intraoperative consultation of head and neck specimens.

Qihui "Jim" Zhai, MD, FCAP

Acknowledgments

My thanks start with Dr. Philip Cagle, the editor-in-chief of the Frozen Section Library Series, not only for his invitation to write this volume, but also for his constructive advice and meticulous editing.

The process of preparing this manuscript reminded me of so many wonderful learning experiences in head and neck pathology. Throughout my residency, fellowship, and academic practices, my career development was nurtured by these outstanding pathologists. Thank you, Drs. Krishnan Unni, Mario Luna, El-Naggar, Alberto Ayala, Jae Ro, and Mary Schwartz.

Collaborative working relationships with head and neck surgeons at the University of Cincinnati have taught me a great deal about what we need to focus on, and their hard work has provided an abundance of interesting cases. Input and feedback from our residents' brilliant young minds aided me in extending the educational scope of this volume.

Above all, I would like to thank my wife Jenny and my daughter Jasmine for their love, understanding, and support.

Contents

Chapter 1
General Considerations

Intraoperative diagnoses of head and neck lesions are extremely important and may provide direct evidence and foundation for the extent of the surgery. However, a frozen section should not be performed unless there will be an immediate impact on intraoperative surgical treatment.

Sometimes, the surgical procedure is not subject to change regardless of what diagnosis a pathologist may render; occasionally, surgeons may want to know the diagnosis intraoperatively for convenience, including more rapid communication with the patient and/or patient's family. In such scenarios, tissue is best saved for permanent evaluation rather than performing a frozen section. The frozen section artifacts, suboptimal histology of the frozen section, pressure for an immediate diagnosis, and lack of ancillary studies at the time of intraoperative consult are among the limitations of the frozen section diagnosis. With better quality histology and additional anxillary studies such as immunohistochemistry, flow cytometry, etc., we may be able to make a more thorough diagnosis on the permanent evaluation. Therefore, frozen sections that are unnecessary for immediate intraoperative therapeutic decisions may waste precious tissue and potentially impact the quality of patient care. A courteous and professional communication with surgeons reiterating these shortcomings of frozen section is prudent.

The following aspects will be addressed in this book. The same format will be used in all the organ-based chapters:

Communications with the surgeon are extremely important. This teamwork will serve in the best interest of the patient. However, to many this may sound like a common-sense suggestion, it cannot be overemphasized in the frozen section laboratory. Oftentimes,

Q.J. Zhai, *Frozen Section Library: Head and Neck*, Frozen Section Library 5, DOI 10.1007/978-0-387-95988-7_1, © Springer Science+Business Media, LLC 2011

we have little clinical information and time is short considering that the patient is anesthetized on the operating table. A direct communication with the surgical colleague is the most reliable and efficient way to understand the history, diagnostic needs, and clinical implications.

Understanding the clinical scenarios, indications, and what information the surgeon needs to know for the particular case to determine the optimal immediate surgical treatment. We do not need to struggle to provide more information than necessary; the consultation we offer should be direct and to the point. The more we say, the more we may need to retract.

Frequent indications requested for frozen section diagnosis in head and neck surgery. Approaches between different institutions and different surgeons may vary. Each organ may have different indications based on the individual patient. However, the following are the major indications: assessment of adequate surgical margins for a known malignant tumor; determination of the nature of the lesion, reactive versus neoplastic; evaluation of the specimen adequacy; or presence of lesional tissue for additional tests, such as flow cytometry, culture, molecular tests, etc.

Handling the specimen appropriately and gross examination. Frozen section starts with gross examination of the specimen. Surgeons know where the areas of concern are; when they label these areas or help orient the specimen personally, it is very helpful to us. Gross appearance of a lesion is most of the time correlated with the microscopic histology. A typical gross appearance will help assure our microscopic conclusion.

Be familiar with the frozen section diagnostic pitfalls and pearls for your differential diagnoses, taking the freezing artifacts into consideration. They are the foundation of an analytical approach to resolve diagnostic issues from each case.

Defer to permanent is a valid option for difficult cases to avoid an irreversible overtreatment. Defer to permanent section is an option for challenging cases; struggling for a diagnosis which might lead to an irreversible consequence is not in the best interests of the patient, surgeon, or pathologist. A malignant diagnosis might result in a wide excision of the primary lesion or a neck node dissection. A reactive atypia induced by previous radiation therapy can be challenging and confusing to us. Being aware of the treatment history of the patient is extremely important; this can help avoid a possible overdiagnosis.

Sometimes, a frozen section diagnosis should not be attempted

1. No immediate surgical implications; a frozen section was performed out of curiosity of the surgeon or for the convenience to discuss with the patient family
2. To establish a primary melanoma or assess the margin of the specimen with previous melanocytic lesions
3. Technically difficult specimen such as heavily ossified tissue
4. Try to establish a firm diagnosis for a specimen with a lymphoid proliferation, since an accurate classification of lymphoma often needs more than just H&E sections. Frozen section may not be able to distinguish a reactive from neoplastic lymphoid process

Chapter 2
Nasal Cavity and Paranasal Sinuses

INTRODUCTION

Included in this chapter are nasal cavities, frontal sinus, ethmoid complex, sphenoid sinus, and maxillary sinuses. These cavities and sinuses are lined by Schneiderian mucosa, consisting of pseudostratified columnar ciliated epithelium with interspersed goblet cells. The roof of the nasal cavity is the cribriform plate, a specific location for olfactory neuroblastoma. The sinonasal Schneiderian (inverted type) papilloma appears to be a precursor of a sinonasal squamous cell carcinoma. Because of the intimate anatomic relationship with the brain, some intracranial lesions/tissues can be seen and the details will be discussed in Chapter 6.

MAJOR DIAGNOSTIC CONSIDERATIONS

- Schneiderian papilloma including inverted, oncocytic, and exophytic patterns. Most inverted papillomas originate from the respiratory mucosa of the lateral nasal wall and paranasal sinuses. Schneiderian papillomas can present with mixed inverted and exophytic patterns.
- Squamous cell carcinoma arising from papilloma
- Nasopharyngeal carcinoma (typical histologic type is lymphoepithelioma-like carcinoma)
- Sinonasal undifferentiated carcinoma
- Fungal ball in the setting of a progressive sinusitis, identification of fungal microorganisms is important; resection of the involved tissue and debridement will be performed.
- Wegener's granulomatosis

Q.J. Zhai, *Frozen Section Library: Head and Neck*, Frozen Section Library 5,
DOI 10.1007/978-0-387-95988-7_2, © Springer Science+Business Media, LLC 2011

- Minor salivary gland tumors do occur in these organs because minor salivary glands exist in the submucosa throughout the aerodigestive tract.
- Possibility of a lymphoma, including B- or T-cell type.

Common Small Round Blue Cell Malignant Tumors in This Area
- Olfactory neuroblastoma/esthesioneuroblastoma
- Rhabdomyosarcoma
- Small cell carcinoma
- Ewing's sarcoma
- Mesenchymal chondrosarcoma
- Lymphoma (except large cell types)

WHAT SURGEONS NEED TO KNOW INTRAOPERATIVELY TO CHOOSE THE OPTIMAL IMMEDIATE SURGICAL MODALITY
- Distinguish benign from malignant lesions
- Establish a differential diagnosis for small blue cell tumors
- Assessment of the resection margins
- Debridement of the necrotic tissue in the presence of inflammation
- Identify the origin of the tissue specimen
- Determine if the lesion is infectious. If granulomata are present, additional fresh and noncontaminated tissue should be requested for culture
- Determine if lymphoid proliferation is present; if yes, then pathologist needs to decide if the tissue is sufficient for additional analysis

SPECIMEN HANDLING AND GROSS DIAGNOSIS
- If a larger resection specimen is presented and the margins are of concern, then orientation and appropriate inking are critical. In some institutions, margins may be obtained from the procedure beds.
- For small biopsies, a smear preparation can be useful before exhausting the tissue by freezing all the fresh tissue, which might be needed for further studies.
- Papillomas may present with some frond-like structures. We should make sure that the sections are oriented to show the surface, so that the growth pattern can be appreciated.

USEFUL DIAGNOSTIC PEARLS
- Changes associated with radiation or chemotherapy should be kept in mind; communication with the surgeon is essential regarding the therapeutic history, since some malignant lesions would receive a preoperative therapy.
- Reviewing previous material when available is very helpful, since many tumor types, each with a wide histologic spectrum, exist in this region.

- Schneiderian papilloma can grow in different patterns, including exophytic, oncocytic, and inverted. Theses papillomas are lined by ciliated respiratory epithelium; they should have more than ten cell layers and central fibrovascular cores holding the finger-like structures. Presence of some mucocytes is indicative of Schneiderian origin. Since they grow downward, inverted papillomas can be challenging to diagnose, and their structure can be complex. Thus, a low power view is more important and allows easier appreciation of the relationship with the surface epithelium (Figs. 2.1 and 2.2).

- Make sure that the complex structure is not misinterpreted as an invasive process. On the other hand, it is not uncommon to see malignant transformation in the keratinized epithelium of an inverted papilloma. In cases like these, inverted papillomas are the precursor lesions. The histologic criteria to evaluate dysplasia arising in a papilloma are cellular disorganization (loss of horizontal arrangement in the superficial layers), cellular immaturity with increased nuclear cytoplasmic ratio, increased mitotic figures, and often atypical mitoses (Fig. 2.3). Sampling the specimen cautiously and sectioning the frozen chuck at multiple levels can be useful to avoid an underdiagnosis.

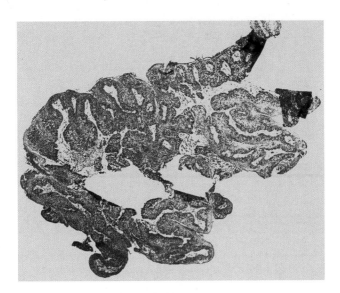

FIG. 2.1 Inverted papilloma low power view. The outer contour of the lesion is the original surface epithelium, and the papillary structures grow downward into the lamina propria by invagination or direct extension into the underlying minor salivary glands forming complex structures.

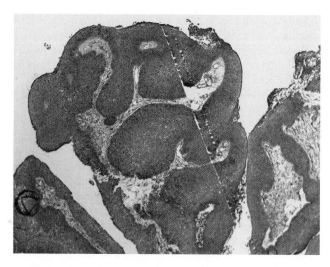

FIG. 2.2 Higher power of the inverted papilloma showing the thickened epithelium with more than ten cell layers. The epithelium shows maturation with no marked cytologic atypia.

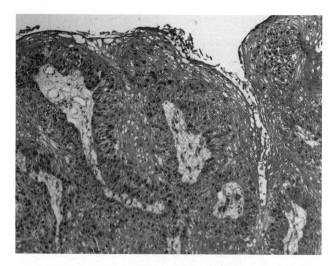

FIG. 2.3 Inverted papilloma with squamous carcinoma in situ, characterized by marked cellular disturbance and nuclear pleomorphism.

- Lymphoepithelioma-like carcinoma still maintains some basic features of carcinoma, such as cohesive tumor cells. In this particular entity, the tumor cells demonstrate a syncytial look and are buried within a lymphoid background (Figs. 2.4 and 2.5). Thus, it can be mistaken for a germinal center, composed of a mixed cellularity.

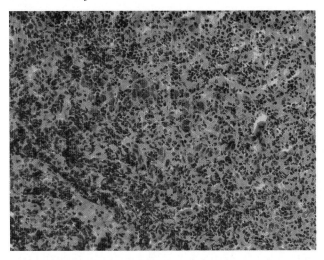

FIG. 2.4 Low power of a lymphoepithelioma-like carcinoma. Nasopharyngeal carcinoma, islands of tumor cells intimately admixed with lymphocytes and plasma cells. Do not confuse the tumor nests with a germinal center.

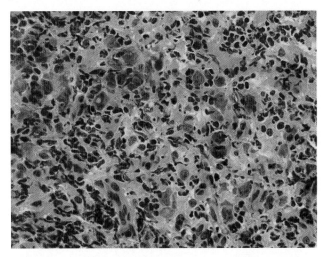

FIG. 2.5 Syncytial carcinoma cells exhibit indistinct cell borders, pale chromatin, and distinct nucleoli while the lymphocytes are mingled within carcinoma cell islands.

- For the small blue cell tumors, there are overlapping histologic features. Most of the time, immunostains are needed to separate them. The lymphoma specimen will show discohesion; small cell carcinoma shows cellular molding; olfactory neuroblastoma is lobulated with a fibrillary matrix/stroma; Ewing's sarcoma tumor cells are so monotonous that individual cells appear to be identical; rhabdomyosarcoma often shows plasmacytoid features. The location of the tumor is critical. If the tumor is from the cribriform plate and shows this morphology, olfactory neuroblastoma should be considered first (Figs. 2.6 and 2.7).

- Mucosal melanoma can be seen and the previous diagnosis might not be available at the time of frozen section. The melanocytic tumor cells are less cohesive than carcinoma cells, but more cohesive than lymphoma cells (Fig. 2.8).

- Geographic necrosis combined with a vasculitis is highly suspicious of Wegener's granulomatosis. Clinical and laboratory tests such as antineutrophil cytoplasmic antibodies (ANCAs) are useful for the diagnosis.

- If a lymphoid proliferation is clinically suspicious, a frozen section may not be necessary, especially when the tissue is scanty; a touch preparation is necessary and it should be made certain that adequate fresh tissue is available. If not, a request for additional fresh tissue should be communicated with the

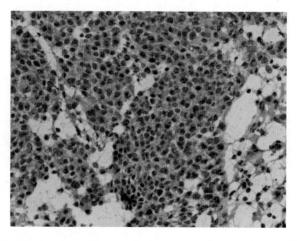

Fig. 2.6 Olfactory neuroblastoma/esthesioneuroblastoma. Nesting/lobular tumor cells with neuroendocrine appearance. The cells are not cohesive.

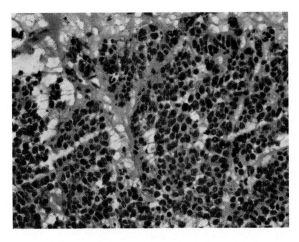

FIG. 2.7 Small cell carcinoma shows nuclear molding and scanty cytoplasm.

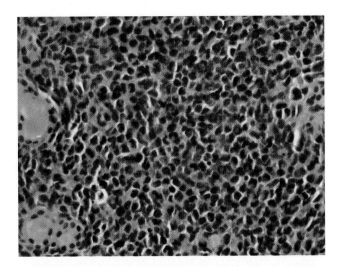

FIG. 2.8 Plasmacytoid cytology and pigment within the tumor cells are indicative of a melanocytic tumor (mucosal melanoma). Although final diagnosis needs ancillary tests such as immunohistochemistry, these histologic features can essentially rule out a lymphoma.

surgeon. It is important to inform the surgeon that this is a lymphoproliferative process; therefore, the surgeon will not chase a clear resection margin (Figs. 2.9 and 2.10).

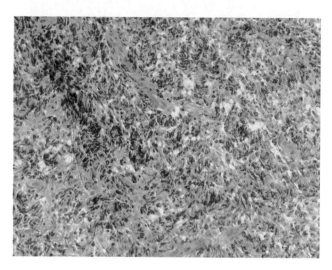

FIG. 2.9 Lymphoma with marked crush artifact. This kind of artifact is most often seen in both small cell carcinoma and lymphoma, since tumor cells from these two entities are fragile.

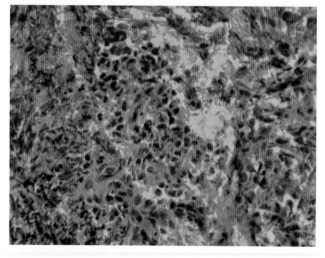

FIG. 2.10 Higher power of a different area with a less distorted histology, tumor cells are discohesive. A possible lymphoma needs to be worked up.

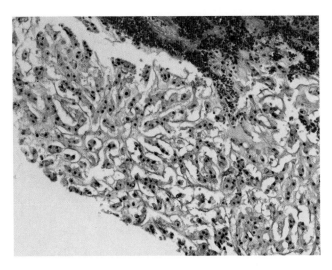

FIG. 2.11 Relatively bland chordoma tumor cells show a lobular configuration in a mucinous background; the tumor cells form typical cord structures mimicking liver plates.

- Chordoma predominantly occurs in the midline of the human body. In the head and neck area, chordomas can involve the spheno-occipital region, including the posterior nasal cavity, sphenoid sinus, nasopharynx, and base of the skull. Low power shows a lobular configuration with mucinous background. Higher power shows relatively bland tumor cells with typical cord-like structures mimicking liver plates (Fig. 2.11).
- Fungal balls can be recognized on frozen section with confidence (Fig. 2.12).

COMMON DIAGNOSTIC PITFALLS
- Extensive fibrosis and granulation tissue with reactive epithelioid endothelial proliferation, which may mimic malignant neoplasm
- Distinction among the small blue cell tumors may require permanent and immunohistochemical studies and should not be attempted on frozen section evaluation
- Reactive hyperplasia of squamous and respiratory epithelia can be difficult to distinguish from papilloma

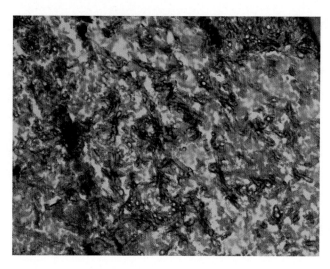

Fɪɢ. 2.12 Fungal ball consisting of septate hyphae with acute-angle branching and features consistent with *Aspergillus.*

Chapter 3
Salivary Glands

INTRODUCTION

Salivary gland tumors are known for their many entities and wide histopathologic spectrum even within any single tumor type. The accurate classification of these entities can be difficult on permanent section, let alone frozen section. Thus, accurate classification of salivary gland tumors on frozen section is not the aim for the intraoperative consultation. Our goal should be to perform an intraoperative consultation for the surgeon that provides enough information to guide the surgical procedure. Understanding the surgical implications of a diagnosis is essential and can make stressful frozen sections less of a struggle. For example, if we appreciate a tumor with an infiltrating border and marked cytologic atypia composed of both squamoid and glandular formations, we may not need to specifically distinguish adenosquamous carcinoma from mucoepidermoid carcinoma, since this distinction will not change the extent of the operational procedure. With this approach, frozen section diagnoses of salivary gland lesions are largely reliable with high sensitivity and specificity, as evidenced by our own experience as well as published data in the literature.

MAJOR DIAGNOSTIC CONSIDERATIONS

Basic demographic information and the typical histologic features of each neoplastic entity are still the foundation of the frozen section interpretation. Salivary glands are divided into major (parotid, submandibular, and sublingual) and minor (intraoral and upper aerodigestive tract submucosa) salivary glands. Differences exist between major and minor salivary glands and their neoplasms in

15

Q.J. Zhai, *Frozen Section Library: Head and Neck*, Frozen Section Library 5, DOI 10.1007/978-0-387-95988-7_3, © Springer Science+Business Media, LLC 2011

the following aspects: anatomy, histology, incidence of different tumors, varying histologic features within the same entity, and potential selection of different surgical procedures. Major salivary gland neoplasms are likely to be benign (roughly 80% for parotid tumors and 50% for submandibular and sublingual tumors) and minor salivary gland tumors are more likely to be malignant (about 20% are benign tumors). In other words, think "benign" first when handling a major salivary gland tumor, and think "malignant" first when handling a minor salivary gland tumor.

Being familiar with the clinical presentation, gross features, diagnostic pearls, and solutions to the pitfalls for the following commonly encountered salivary gland tumors will help us provide accurate intraoperative consultations in our daily practice:

- *Pleomorphic adenoma* (PA, mixed tumor) (Figs. 3.1–3.16)
- *Warthin tumor* (Figs. 3.17–3.20)
- *Mucoepidermoid carcinoma.* Mucoepidermoid carcinoma not only occurs in adults, but may also occur in children. It is the most frequent malignant salivary gland tumor in children. The key is to recognize the cystic structures lined by mucocytes, squamoid cells and intermingled with intermediate cells (Figs. 3.21–3.27)
- *Acinic cell adenocarcinoma* (Figs. 3.28–3.30)

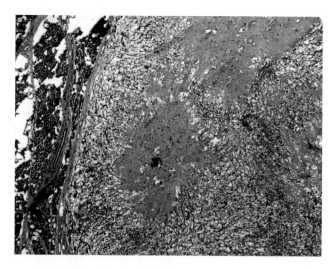

Fig. 3.1   PA: Low power picture demonstrates a fibrous capsule, interfacing between tumor and the abutting benign salivary gland tissue. This view is predominantly myxoid with hypocellular myoepithelial component.

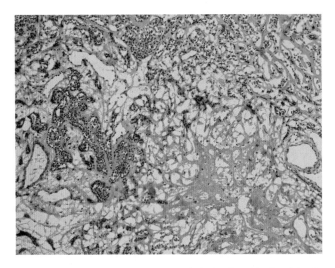

FIG. 3.2   PA: Dual cell differentiation: epithelial cells with glandular formation admixed with myoepithelial cells merged in a myxoid matrix.

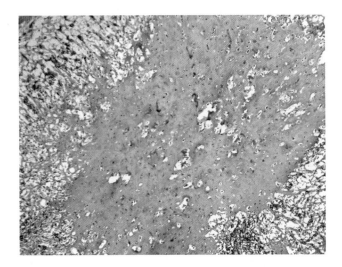

FIG. 3.3   PA: Chondroid/cartilaginous material is diagnostic of a PA.

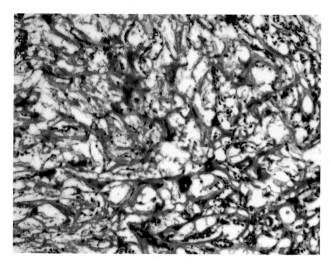

FIG. 3.4 **PA:** Myoepithelial cell melting into the myxoid matrix with a submerged appearance within the myxoid matrix/stroma.

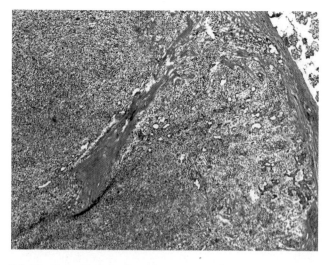

FIG. 3.5 **PA:** Myoepithelial cell predominance with very little epithelial cell tubular and glandular structures in the upper right area.

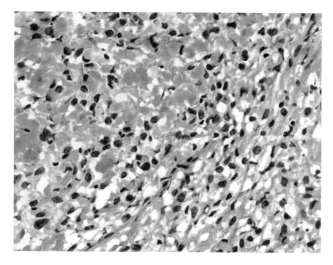

FIG. 3.6 **PA:** Myoepithelial cells with spindle and plasmacytoid appearances and their products, basement material.

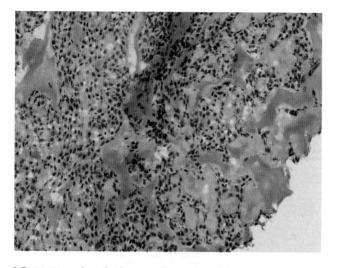

FIG. 3.7 **PA:** Vaguely cribriform configuration with a myxoid stroma mimics adenoid cystic carcinoma. A constellation of features needs to be considered to separate these two entities, including the tumor growth border, tumor growth architecture, and perineural invasion.

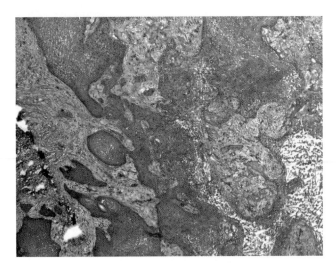

FIG. 3.8 **PA** with reactive changes induced by previous FNA. Squamous metaplasia induced by previous FNA, mimicking a squamous cell carcinoma. The FNA procedure is a widely applied diagnostic tool. The procedure alone may generate reactive changes ranging from infarction to squamous cell metaplasia. Being aware of the prefrozen section FNA is essential. This can help us to correlate the FNA findings with frozen section while simultaneously warning us of the potential artifacts induced by the procedure, aiding us to avoid the diagnostic trap.

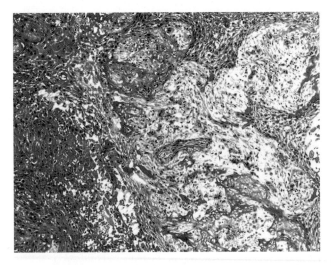

FIG. 3.9 **PA**: An area of squamous metaplasia with a pseudoinvasive pattern mimicking a squamous cell carcinoma.

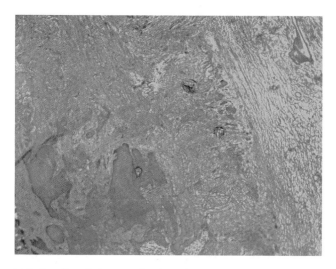

FIG. 3.10 PA: The whole view of a PA with squamous metaplasia; note that the upper right periphery of the tumor shows typical features of a PA.

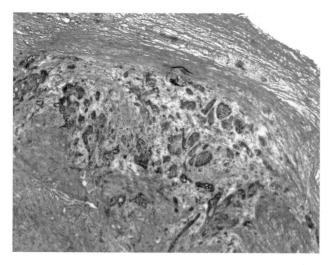

FIG. 3.11 PA: Higher power view of the typical PA histology.

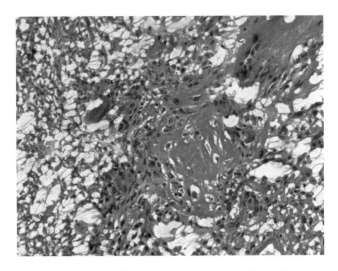

FIG. 3.12   PA with tissue infarction/necrosis and reactive atypia.

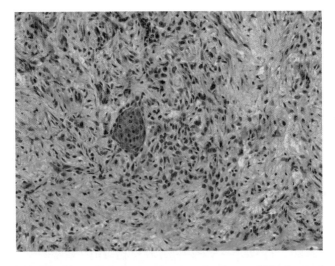

FIG. 3.13   PA with marked reactive change and a cluster of bland metaplastic squamous cells.

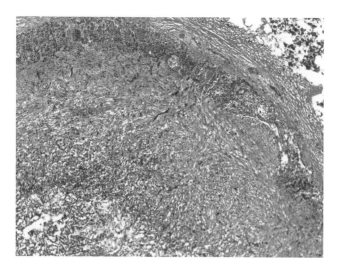

FIG. 3.14 The overview demonstrates PA features at the right upper periphery and the infarction as well as the reactive changes in the center.

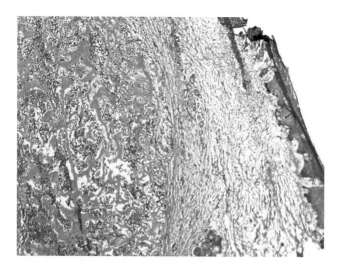

FIG. 3.15 A minor salivary gland PA is well demarcated, but not encapsulated.

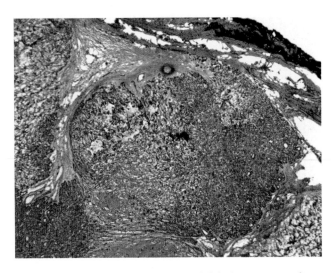

Fig. 3.16 A recurrent PA demonstrates multilobular pattern, a diagnostic pitfall for invasion.

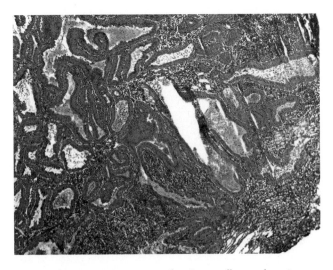

Fig. 3.17 Warthin tumor: Low power showing papillary and cystic structures lined by oncocytic epithelial cells and dense stromal lymphoid tissue with a germinal center appearance.

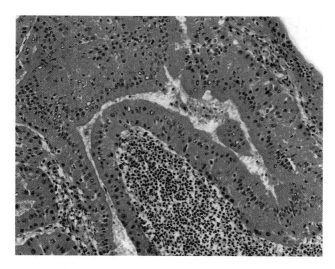

FIG. 3.18 Warthin tumor: Higher power showing the two cell layer of oncocytic cells lining papillae and the surrounding dense lymphoid stroma.

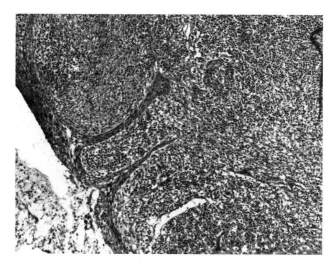

FIG. 3.19 Squamous metaplasia may be misinterpreted as a squamous cell carcinoma within a Warthin tumor.

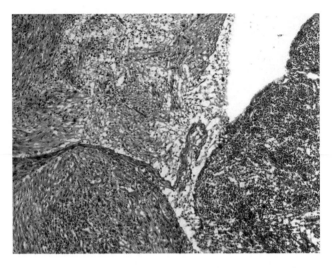

Fig. 3.20 Squamous metaplasia adjacent to the typical Warthin tumor cells, confirming the metaplastic nature.

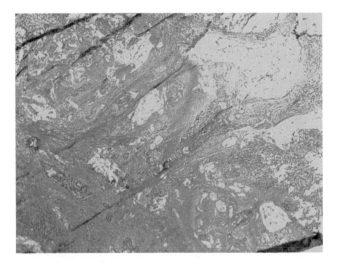

Fig. 3.21 Mucoepidermoid carcinoma: Low power demonstrates a cystic structure with a pushing border pattern and pools of mucus extravasation.

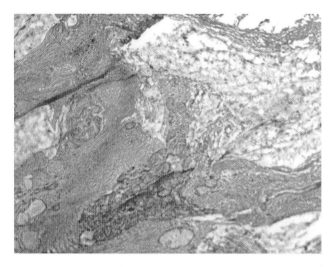

FIG. 3.22 Mucoepidermoid carcinoma: Epidermoid cells, mucocytes, and intermediate cells are the three major components for this entity.

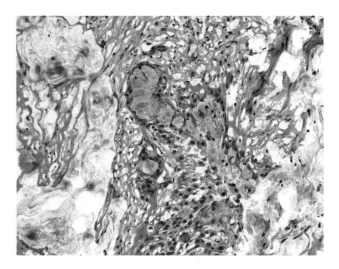

FIG. 3.23 Mucoepidermoid carcinoma: Higher power of the mucocytes and epidermoid cells with mucus.

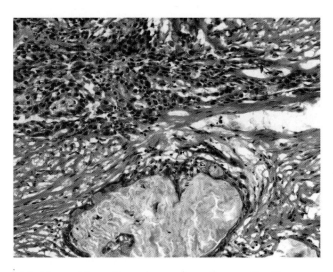

F<small>IG</small>. 3.24   Mucoepidermoid carcinoma: A smaller cyst lined by mucocytes and adjacent pocket of solid squamoid area admixed with intermediate cells.

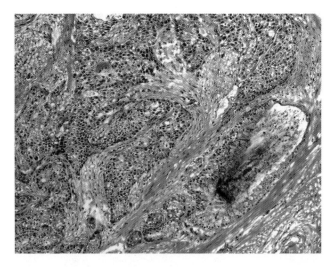

F<small>IG</small>. 3.25   An example of a higher grade of mucoepidermoid carcinoma evidenced by more solid areas. The grading system considers cystic component, perineural invasion, necrosis, number of mitosis, and anaplasia.

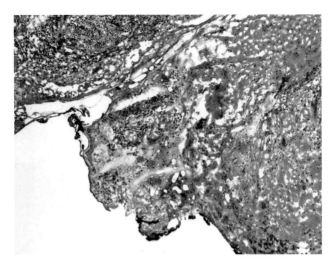

FIG. 3.26   Mucoepidermoid carcinoma was transected at the inked resection margin.

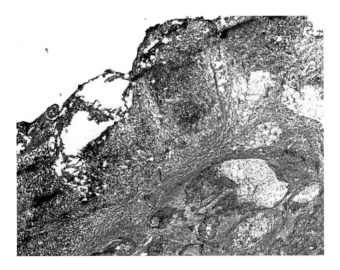

FIG. 3.27   Mucoepidermoid carcinoma: Another resection margin is negative of tumor. The distance was measured and communicated to the surgeon.

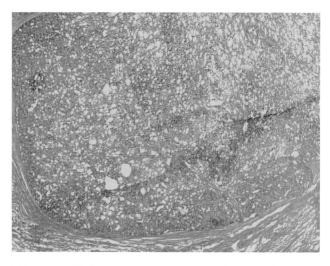

Fɪɢ. 3.28 Acinic cell adenocarcinoma: Low power shows a well-circumscribed growth pattern and areas of acinar appearance at the bottom.

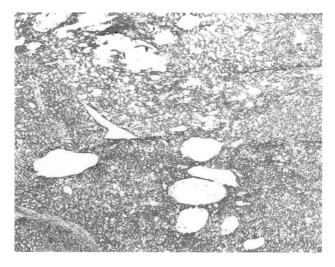

Fɪɢ. 3.29 Different patterns of acinic cell adenocarcinoma, micro- and microcystic structures.

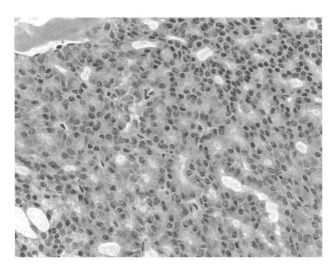

FIG. 3.30 High power of acinic cell carcinoma with deceptively benign appearing tumor cells. Occasionally, it is difficult to be sure that this is indeed a neoplastic process. The pearl is that in acinic cell adenocarcinoma the lobular architecture is effaced and the benign ducts and/or tubules are absent. The tumor is composed of similar cells with granular cytoplasm.

- *Adenoid cystic carcinoma* (Figs. 3.31–3.41)
- *Polymorphous low-grade adenocarcinoma* (PLGA). By its name, the tumor is composed of different growth patterns including solid, cribriform, streaming, cystic, trabecular, tubular, and glandular. "Low-grade" is used for this entity due to its bland look of the tumor cells. It is histologically an adenocarcinoma because of its infiltrating nature (Figs. 3.42–3.51)
- *Myoepithelial carcinoma* (Figs. 3.52–3.54)
- *Oncocytoma* (Figs. 3.55 and 3.56)
- *Adenocarcinoma, NOS* (not otherwise specified) (Figs. 3.57 and 3.58)
- *Sebaceous lymphadenoma*. Salivary gland tissue contains rich lymphoid tissue. Sometimes, the lymphoid tissue is part of the tumor, such as Warthin tumor and this entity (Figs. 3.59 and 3.60)
- *Carcinoma ex-pleomorphic adenoma (Ca. ex-PA)*. We need to see a typical PA and then a carcinoma arising from this PA, before such a diagnosis should be rendered. The carcinoma component can be any histologic type of salivary gland tumor,

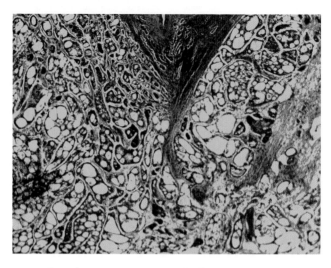

Fɪɢ. 3.31 Adenoid cystic carcinoma: Cribriform and tubulocystic growth pattern.

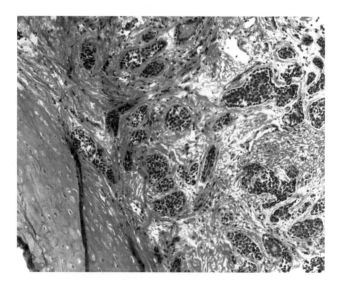

Fɪɢ. 3.32 Adenoid cystic carcinoma: Infiltrating growth pattern involving the cartilage.

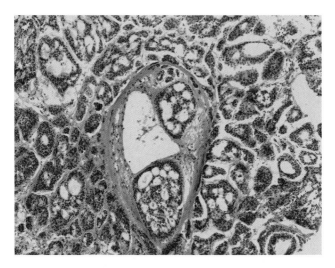

Fig. 3.33 Adenoid cystic carcinoma: Swiss cheese cribriform growth pattern.

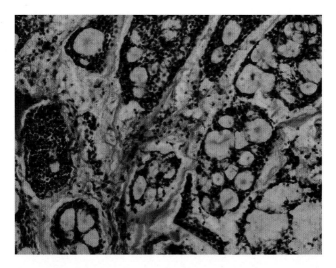

Fig. 3.34 Adenoid cystic carcinoma: The pseudoglandular formation (adenoid rather than adeno-) is evinced by the opening of the "gland lumens" and connections between the spaces within the stroma sharing the same gray/bluish mucinous basement material.

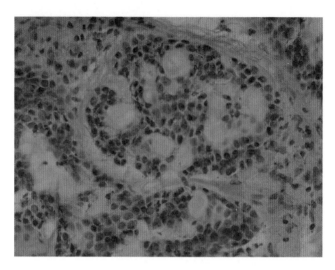

FIG. 3.35 Adenoid cystic carcinoma: High magnification demonstrates the cell details; the tumor cells are small and hyperchromatic without marked pleomorphism or necrosis, or brisk mitosis.

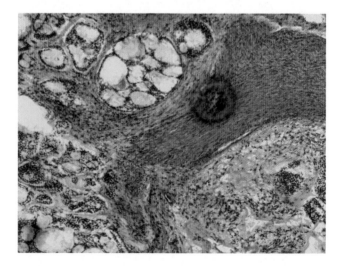

FIG. 3.36 Adenoid cystic carcinoma: A thick nerve bundle was surrounded by the tumor.

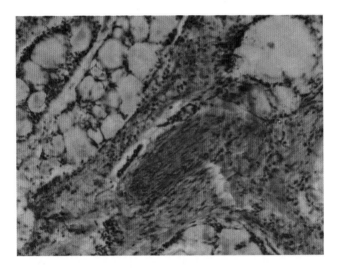

FIG. 3.37 Adenoid cystic carcinoma: Another area of perineural invasion, a typical finding for this tumor.

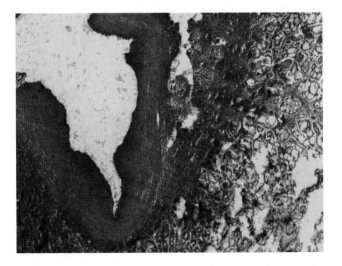

FIG. 3.38 Adenoid cystic carcinoma: Tumor clusters invading into the wall of an artery (mid upper).

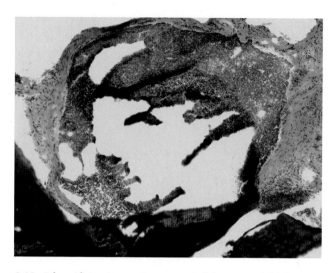

FIG. 3.39   Adenoid cystic carcinoma: A solid area involving the bone. The necrosis and solid pattern suggest a higher grade of adenoid cystic carcinoma.

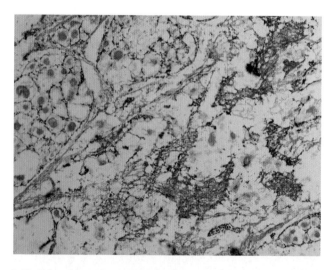

FIG. 3.40   Adenoid cystic carcinoma: The myxoid stroma is also part of the spectrum. Do not confuse this histology with that of a PA. The solution is to search for histologically malignant features such as an infiltrating growth pattern, perineural invasion, etc.

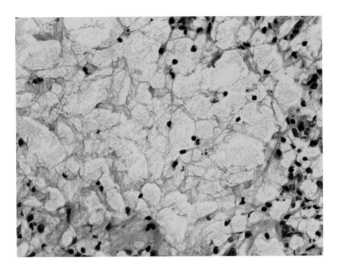

FIG. 3.41 Adenoid cystic carcinoma: As a comparison to Fig. 3.4, the myoepithelial cells stand out from the myxoid matrix in adenoid cystic carcinoma. This is one of the useful diagnostic parameters to separate a PA from adenoid cystic carcinoma.

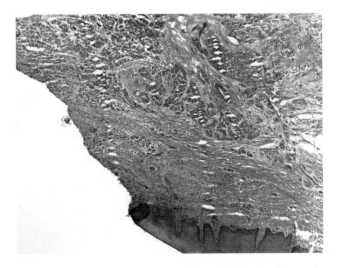

FIG. 3.42 **PLGA**: Low power of the tumor in the hard palate without a capsule and not well circumscribed either.

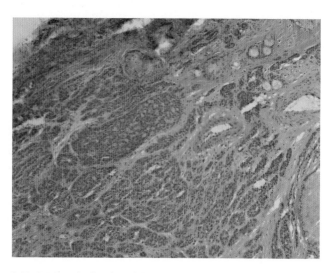

FIG. 3.43 **PLGA:** The border of the tumor invades into the adjacent benign minor salivary glands. There are cribriform and trabecular growth patterns in this field.

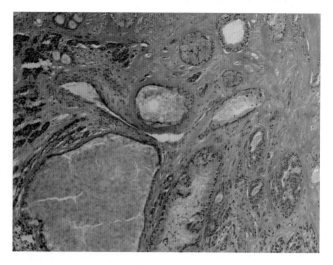

FIG. 3.44 **PLGA:** A higher magnification of the invasive component in between the benign mucinous minor salivary glands.

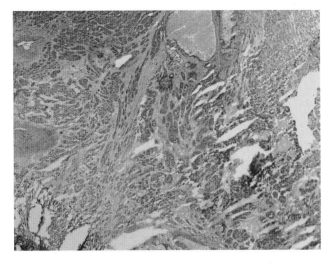

FIG. 3.45 **PLGA:** Different growth patterns of tumor within one field.

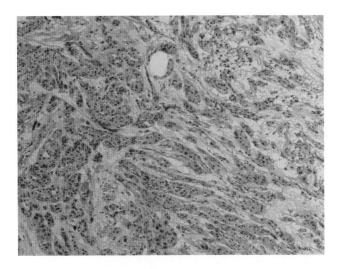

FIG. 3.46 **PLGA:** Trabecular, cystic, and streaming patterns within one field.

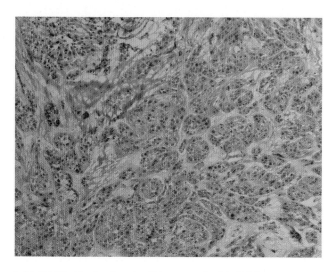

Fig. 3.47 **PLGA:** Predominant solid pattern in this field.

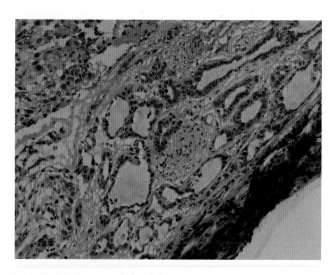

Fig. 3.48 **PLGA:** Cystic and glandular patterns.

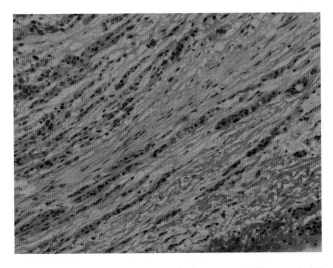

FIG. 3.49 **PLGA:** Area with a streaming look to it, reminding us of a lobular breast carcinoma.

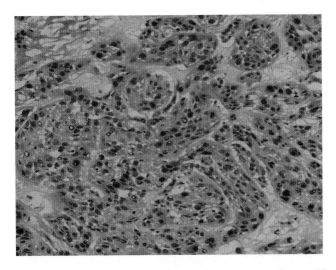

FIG. 3.50 **PLGA:** High power of the cytology, tumor cells are bland, monotonous and have vesicular nuclei. These cytologic features are useful to separate this entity from adenoid cystic carcinoma.

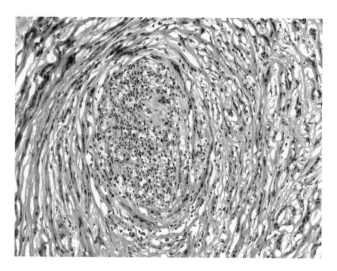

Fig. 3.51 **PLGA:** Perineural invasion is very helpful establishing a diagnosis of malignancy, since the cytology for this entity is usually bland. The pattern is that of an onion ring with tumor cells surrounding the nerve in a laminated manner.

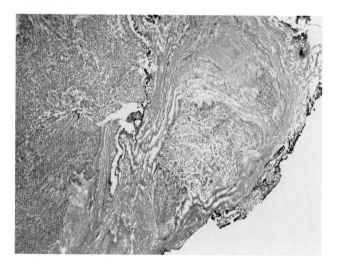

Fig. 3.52 Myoepithelial carcinoma: Low power picture demonstrates an infiltrating tumor growth border, an important malignant diagnostic feature.

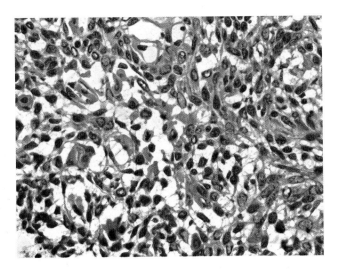

F<small>IG</small>. 3.53 **Myoepithelial carcinoma:** Tumor is composed of spindle and plasmacytoid myoepithelial cells with marked cytologic atypia and mitotic figures.

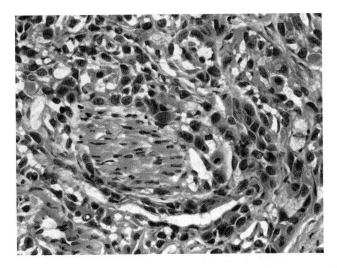

F<small>IG</small>. 3.54 **Myoepithelial carcinoma:** Perineural invasion, a very useful histologic feature for a malignant diagnosis, is responsible for local recurrence and distant metastasis. This feature is often seen in adenoid cystic carcinoma as well.

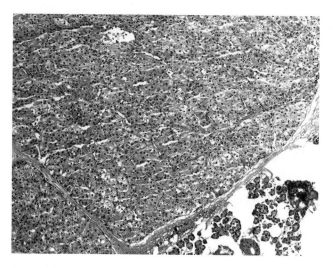

FIG. 3.55 Oncocytoma: Encapsulated oncocytic tumor with no obvious cytologic atypia.

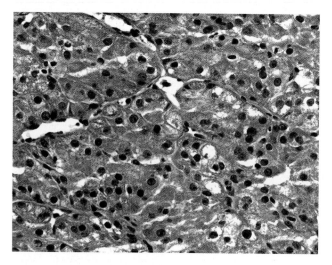

FIG. 3.56 Oncocytoma: High power shows the organoid tumor cells with eosinophilic granular cytoplasm and noticeable nucleoli.

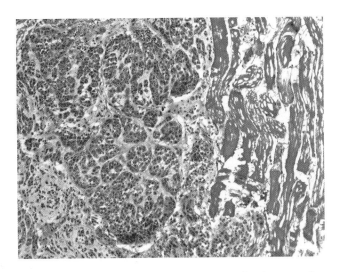

FIG. 3.57 Adenocarcinoma, NOS: Lower power showing an adenocarcinoma involving skeletal muscle. This histology is not specific for any well-defined tumor within salivary gland. For this reason, "not otherwise specified" is used to describe this type of adenocarcinoma.

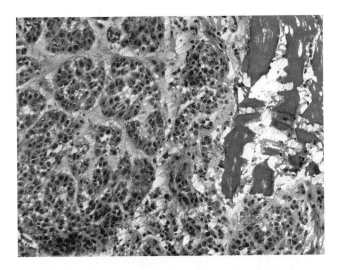

FIG. 3.58 Adenocarcinoma, NOS: High power showing malignant cells with prominent nucleoli and gland formation. While at the frozen section, based on the specimen provided, a diagnosis of adenocarcinoma, NOS was rendered, which was most appropriate. The subsequent resection of the parotid shows a ca. ex-PA.

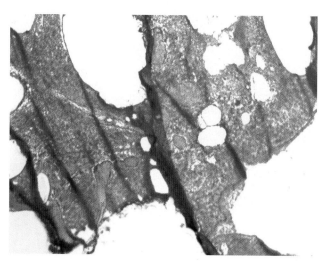

FIG. 3.59 Sebaceous lymphadenoma. Low power view, a multicystic lesion with lymphoid cells in between.

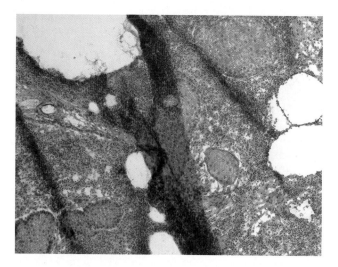

FIG. 3.60 Sebaceous lymphadenoma. High power, sebaceous component is obvious. The major difference between sebaceous lymphadenoma with lymphadenoma is that the latter is lacking a sebaceous component.

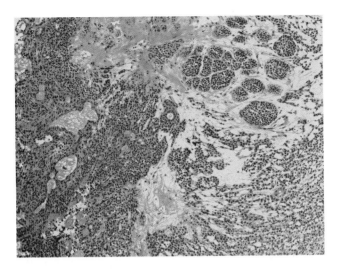

Fɪɢ. 3.61   Ca. ex-PA: *Left part* of the picture: there is a typical PA histology; *right upper quadrant* is an adenoid cystic carcinoma with an appearance of solid pattern.

including adenocarcinoma, squamous carcinoma, adenoid cystic carcinoma, epithelial–myoepithelial carcinoma, polymorphous low-grade adenocarcinoma, salivary duct carcinoma, etc. In this particular case, there is an adenoid cystic carcinoma arising from a PA (Figs. 3.61–3.63)

- *Salivary duct carcinoma.* If the histology reminds you of a high-grade breast ductal carcinoma in situ with comedo necrosis, and the lesion is from salivary gland, it is likely to be a salivary duct carcinoma (Figs. 3.64 and 3.65)

A benign diagnosis such as PA in a parotid gland will limit the resection to superficial lobectomy and spare the facial nerve. If misdiagnosed as a malignancy upon frozen section, the facial nerve might be sacrificed by a wider excision or total parotidectomy, and the quality of the patient's life will be significantly impacted.

Another major indication for frozen section is to determine if the tumor has been completely excised; in other words, whether the resection margin is free of tumor or not. Positive margins are defined by the transection of tumor cells. We can provide the distance from the tumor to the resection margin (tissue shrinks significantly after removal from the human body, especially so for the mucosa).

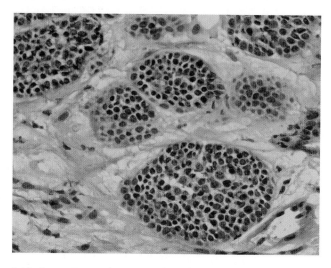

FIG. 3.62 Ca. ex-PA: Higher power of the adenoid cystic carcinoma. The tumor cells are relatively small and darkly stained, typical cytology for an adenoid cystic carcinoma.

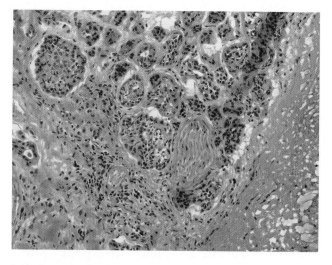

FIG. 3.63 Ca. ex-PA: A separate area of the same case (Fig. 3.62), there is perineural invasion. Perineural invasion is a frequent finding in adenoid cystic carcinoma, although not pathognomonic.

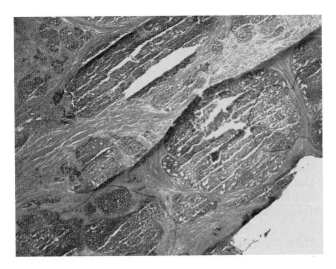

FIG. 3.64 Salivary duct carcinoma with infiltrating, and yet maintaining a ductal growth pattern.

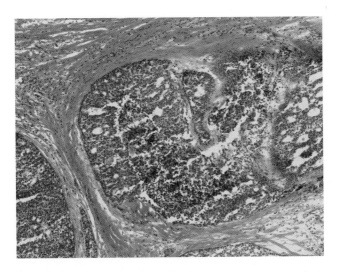

FIG. 3.65 If this picture is said to be obtained from a breast lesion, it would be reasonable to call it a ductal carcinoma in situ, cribriform growth pattern, with comedo necrosis. In this case, the histologic pattern is photographed from a salivary duct carcinoma.

WHAT SURGEONS NEED TO KNOW INTRAOPERATIVELY TO CHOOSE THE OPTIMAL IMMEDIATE SURGICAL MODALITY

- Determine the lesion's nature, such as neoplastic, inflammatory, or congenital
- Determine tumor type (benign vs. malignant), especially when preoperative fine needle aspirate (FNA) was not diagnostic
- Confirmation of previous "suspicious for malignancy" FNA results
- Evaluate surgical resection margins and presence of perineural invasion
- Differentiate primary versus metastatic lesions
- Determine the grade of a malignancy to decide the extent of surgical procedure
- Evaluation of lymph nodes to differentiate metastatic disease from a primary lesion

SPECIMEN HANDLING AND GROSS DIAGNOSIS

The first step of the frozen section diagnosis is to handle the specimen appropriately.

- Make sure the orientation is correct, since this is important if one or more of the resection margins is involved with the tumor. A stitch or orientation by the surgeon is very helpful. Ink the specimen with dedicated colors for orientation.
- Bread-loaf the specimen and expose the cut surface of the lesion. The gross impression is very important. Be sure to note the tumor size, growth pattern at the border, consistency/texture, color, and presence or absence of necrosis.
- An experienced pathologist relies heavily on this technique; by this point, a short list of differential diagnoses should be formed.
- In combination with the patient's sex, age, and the location of the lesion, the list of diagnostic possibilities will have become even shorter. The final microscopic diagnosis is often consistent with the gross impression.

Here are some typical gross features of the most common tumors in salivary gland (Figs. 3.66–3.73):

- A well-circumscribed tumor with cartilaginous appearance located in the parotid gland has a high likelihood of being a PA.
- An infiltrative tumor with a fleshy appearance is highly suggestive of a malignant tumor.
- A cystic lesion with daughter satellites should remind us of a mucoepidermoid carcinoma.
- A cystic brown to tan color lesion with papillae and yellowish fluid is highly suggestive of a Warthin tumor.
- An oncocytic tumor typically shows brown/mahogany color, similar to oncocytic tumors arising in other organs.

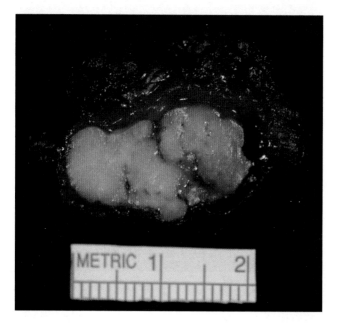

FIG. 3.66 A typical pleomorphic adenoma with well-demarcated tumor border. More diagnostically, the glittering appearance is highly indicative of chondroid/ cartilage differentiation, which is one of the reliable histologic parameters for this entity (Courtesy of Dr. Jun Zhang).

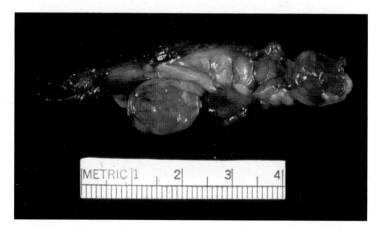

FIG. 3.67 Warthin tumor is characterized by an encapsulated, tan-brown, round to oval tumor mass (Courtesy of Dr. Jun Zhang).

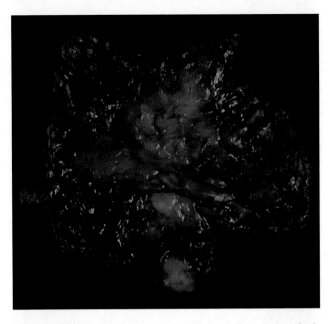

FIG. 3.68 Mucoepidermoid carcinoma is not well circumscribed with satellite nodules. Microscopic review demonstrates an intermediate grade carcinoma. A low-grade tumor should demonstrate more cystic components (Courtesy of Dr. Jun Zhang).

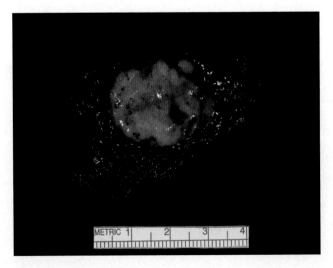

FIG. 3.69 A relatively well-circumscribed main tumor with an adjacent tumor satellite. The cut surface is whitish and fleshy, which is usually a gross appearance of a malignant process. This is an example of acinic cell adencarcinoma. (Courtesy of Dr. Jun Zhang).

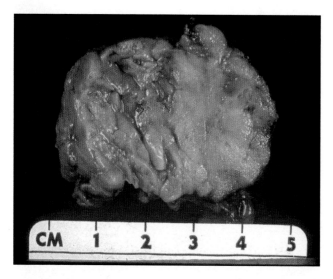

FIG. 3.70 The gross appearance of this adenoid cystic carcinoma is infiltrating and fleshy. There is no clear separation between the benign salivary gland (at the *left of the picture*) and the carcinoma component (Courtesy of Dr. Jun Zhang).

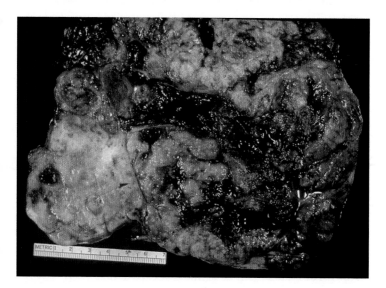

FIG. 3.71 This is a representation of a high-grade malignancy, evidenced by the extensive necrosis and hemorrhage. Careful sectioning demonstrates the coexistence of a carcinoma and a typical pleomorphic adenoma, from which the carcinoma is arising from (Courtesy of Dr. Jun Zhang).

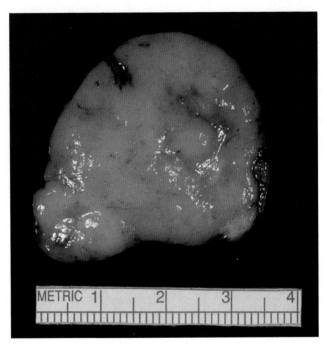

FIG. 3.72 Homogeneous, whitish, as well as a fish–flesh appearance, which is a typical gross picture for a lymphoma (Courtesy of Dr. Jun Zhang).

USEFUL DIAGNOSTIC PEARLS

The following diagnostic pearls have been proven very useful and practical. If used appropriately, we can address most of the diagnostic dilemmas in the frozen section laboratory.

Tumor Growth Borders

Evaluation of the interface between the tumor and the abutting benign salivary gland tissue is very important. This is one of the major diagnostic parameters in distinguishing benign from malignant neoplasms in salivary gland tumors. A tumor with an invasive growth pattern is a malignant process until proven otherwise. On the other hand, a tumor with a clear demarcation with or without a capsule is most likely to be either a benign or a low-grade tumor such as acinic cell carcinoma. Therefore, the specimen should be sampled such that the tumor border can be evaluated. A low-grade malignant tumor which may present as "well circumscribed" is the mucoepidermoid carcinoma.

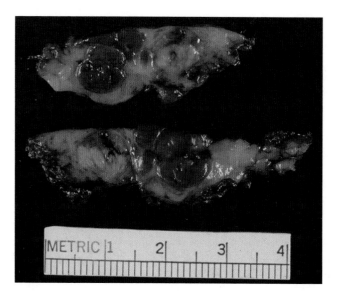

F<small>IG.</small> 3.73 Mahogany in color and well-circumscribed nodules are typical for oncocytoma (Courtesy of Dr. Jun Zhang).

Mostly, it contains several cystic structures lined by mucocytes with intervening squamoid and intermediate cells. The cystic components are invasive in nature; however, they have a pushing border. A mixed tumor occurring in the minor salivary glands is not encapsulated as in the parotid gland, but still maintains a well-demarcated, noninvasive border.

Number of Cell Types

Many salivary gland tumors are composed of more than one cell type including epithelial, myoepithelial cells and/or lymphocytes. The majority of such tumors are PA, adenoid cystic carcinoma, mucoepidermoid carcinoma, epithelial–myoepithelial carcinoma, and Warthin tumor. Single cell type tumors include acinic cell adenocarcinoma, myoepithelioma, adenocarcinoma, NOS, onco-cytoma, polymorphous low-grade adenocarcinoma, salivary duct carcinoma, lymphoma, etc.

Cytologic Atypia

Most of the time, marked cytological atypia is sufficient for the diagnosis of a malignancy. Examples include ca. ex-PA and dediffer-entiation of a lower grade salivary gland tumor. Any type of malig-nancy of salivary gland can be seen in ca. ex-PA, such as salivary duct carcinoma, adenoid cystic carcinoma, squamous carcinoma, adenocarcinoma, etc.

Perineural Invasion
Presence of perineural invasion is another major diagnostic parameter for a malignant neoplasm. It is most frequently seen in adenoid cystic carcinoma and polymorphous low-grade adenocarcinoma. Identification of perineural invasion is reassuring for a diagnosis of malignant tumor.

Interaction Between Epithelial Cells and Stromal Cells
Pleomorphic adenoma is a differential diagnosis for many tumor entities in the salivary gland, especially adenoid cystic carcinoma and polymorphous low-grade adenocarcinoma. This is due to the many overlapping histologic features. The correct diagnosis is imperative because their therapeutic and prognostic implications are dramatically different. Both pleomorphic adenoma and adenoid cystic carcinoma show myoepithelial cells intimately admixed with the myxoid matrix. However, mixed tumors show a more intimate relation; the myoepithelial cells look like they are swimming in a pool of myxoid material. In other words, the myoepithelial cells are merged into the myxoid stroma and are less obviously appreciated. In contrast, the myoepithelial cells in adenoid cystic carcinoma distinctly stand out against the myxoid pool.

Identification of Chondroid and/or Cartilaginous Material
The identification of chondroid and/or cartilaginous material is diagnostic of a PA, since there is no such histologic finding in other entities on the list of differential diagnoses, such as adenoid cystic carcinoma and polymorphous low-grade adenocarcinoma.

Defer to Permanent Is a Valid Option
With various histologic tumor types and mixed growth patterns, a precise diagnosis relying on frozen section might be difficult. Sometimes, it might not be an easy job to tell a benign from a malignant tumor. Deferring to permanent section is a reasonable option for challenging cases. An overcall diagnosis which might lead to an irreversible overtreatment is not in the best interests of the patient, surgeon, or pathologist. A mutual understanding/communication about the limitations and risks with the surgeon is essential in this scenario. Permanent sections will provide a much better morphology and the opportunity to utilize immunohistochemistry,

especially for the cellular differentiation of epithelial cells and/or myoepithelial cells.

COMMON DIAGNOSTIC PITFALLS

- PA, as indicated by its name, can demonstrate a wide histologic spectrum. The tumor may show predominantly myxoid areas with very low cellularity, different growth patterns within the tumor, different combinations of epithelial and myoepithelial cells, hypercellularity, and sometimes cytologic atypia. When these features are encountered, a constellation of parameters should be considered and the above diagnostic pearls should be applied.
- Procedure-induced effect within a benign lesion such as infarction/necrosis and squamous metaplasia within a PA due to previous FNA biopsy may mimic squamous cell carcinoma.
- Cribriform structures in PA can mimic an adenoid cystic carcinoma.
- Recurrent PA can present as multilobular nodules, which can be misdiagnosed as an invasive process.
- Presence of mucin can be misinterpreted as mucocytes. A pool of mucin might represent mucus extravasation and a hunt for mucocytes is justified before a diagnosis of mucoepidermoid carcinoma is rendered.
- Evaluating lymph nodes for lymphoma requires a hematopathology workup. Some pathologists may feel compelled to provide a final diagnosis of lymphoma on the frozen section, but this should be avoided in the setting of a lymphoproliferative process. Currently, flow cytometry and/or molecular technologies are necessary for the classification of lymphomas. The major reason surgeons request frozen sections in this setting is that they need to know if the tissue sample will be diagnostic and sufficient for later, more advanced tests. Therefore, an attempt to accurately classify the lesion using frozen section is not only unnecessary but potentially misleading. Communication with the surgeon is essential when there is a suspicion of lymphoma. Fresh tissue should be sent for flow cytometry in an appropriate medium. After exposure to formalin, the tissue will no longer be amenable to flow cytometry testing.

Chapter 4
Oral Cavity, Pharynx, and Larynx

INTRODUCTION

In this chapter, we discuss issues frequently encountered in the oral cavity (including buccal mucosa and tongue), pharynx (oropharynx, nasopharynx, and hypopharynx including the base of tongue, tonsils, soft palate, and uvula), and larynx (including supraglottis, glottis, and subglottis). We lump these organs together not only because of their anatomic proximicity, but also because of the commonality between lesions seen in these organs. Another shared characteristic is that the pathologic assessment of precursor lesions is similar throughout the upper aerodigestive tract (UADT).

The vast majority of the frozen sections requested from head and neck surgeons are for the evaluation of the surgical margins. Most of the time, the tumors are epithelial in origin and the main body of the cases are squamous cell carcinoma. Therefore, being familiar with the possible mucosal lesions – namely hyperplasia, reactive atypia, dysplasia, carcinoma in situ, or invasive carcinoma – is extremely important (Figs. 4.1–4.29).

EPITHELIAL PRECURSOR LESIONS

Evaluation of squamous epithelium to identify the presence or absence of dysplasia is a task a surgical pathologist frequently has to tackle in daily practice. Criteria used to assess uterine cervical dysplasia have been well defined and widely accepted. The cervical dysplasia criterion mainly relies on the thickness of involvement by the dysplastic cells: namely, mild dysplasia up to the lower one third, moderate dysplasia two thirds, and severe full

Q.J. Zhai, *Frozen Section Library: Head and Neck*, Frozen Section Library 5, DOI 10.1007/978-0-387-95988-7_4, © Springer Science+Business Media, LLC 2011

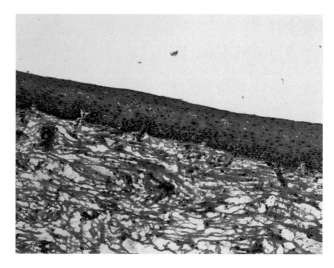

Fig. 4.1   Normal squamous epithelium.

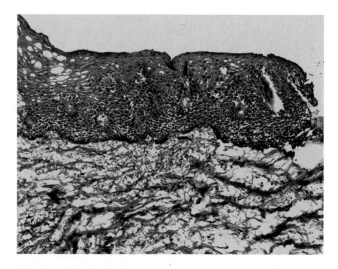

Fig. 4.2   Hyperplasic epithelium, with an increased number of the cell layers. The architecture is not distorted and the cells are not atypical.

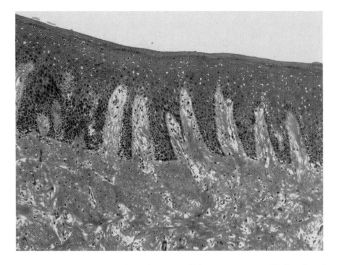

FIG. 4.3 Reactive atypia with architectural distortion, no cellular dysplasia.

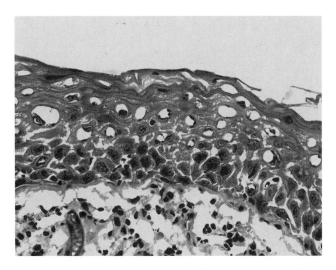

FIG. 4.4 Mild squamous dysplasia. No significant architectural distortion and dysplastic cells confined to the lower third of the epithelium, predominantly in the basal and parabasal areas.

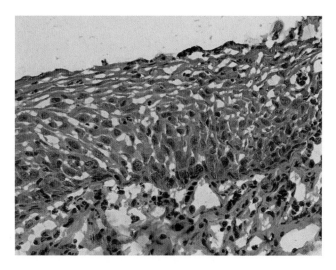

FIG. 4.5 Moderate squamous dysplasia. No significant architectural distortion; dysplastic cells involve up to the mid-third of the epithelium.

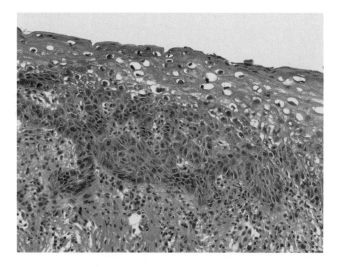

FIG. 4.6 Severe dysplasia. Marked architectural disturbance reaches the mid-third of the epithelium and the cytologic atypia is marked. This is the histology that we need to upgrade from moderate to severe dysplasia.

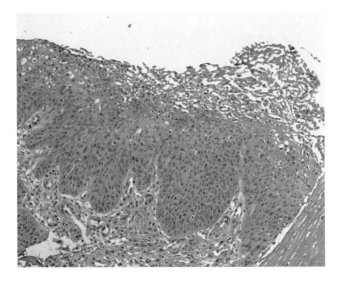

Fig. 4.7 Severe squamous dysplasia with similar features as Fig. 4.6.

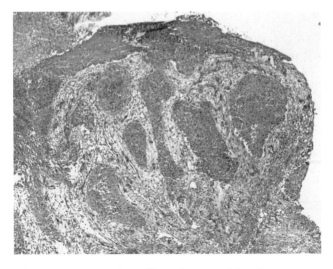

Fig. 4.8 Invasive squamous cell carcinoma arising from an area of "moderate dysplasia", which is not uncommon in the precursor lesions of UADT. This is the histologic rationale to upgrade "moderate dysplasia" to "severe dysplasia".

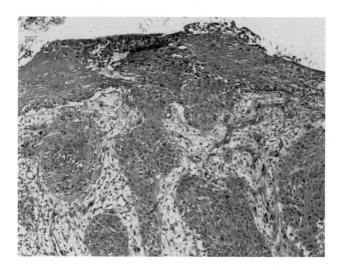

Fig. 4.9   Higher power of Fig. 4.8.

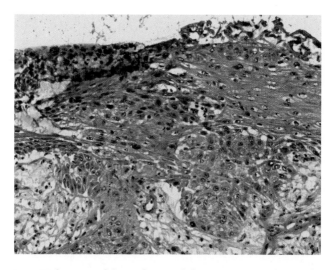

Fig. 4.10   High power of the surface epithelium in Fig. 4.8. There is marked architectural disturbance of the epithelium; however, the dysplastic cells do not reach the very top. A diagnosis of severe squamous dysplasia can be made and a full thickness involvement by dysplasia is not required.

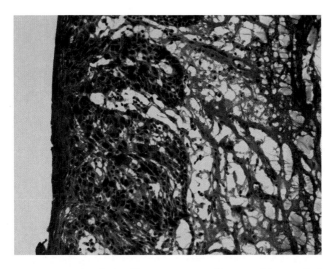

FIG. 4.11 Severe dysplasia. There is no significant architectural disturbance; while the dysplastic cells reach the upper two thirds of the full thickness.

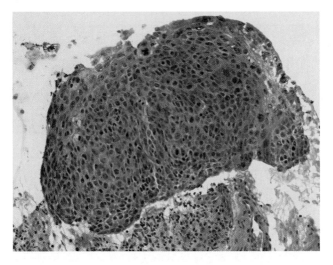

FIG. 4.12 Squamous carcinoma in situ. There is no significant architectural disturbance; while the dysplastic cells involve the full thickness.

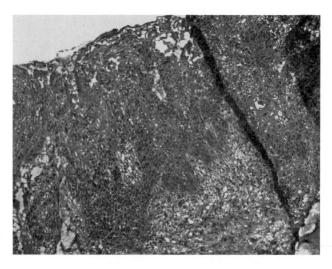

FIG. 4.13 Squamous cell carcinoma in situ with highly distorted architecture and areas of possible microinvasion (at *right lower corner*).

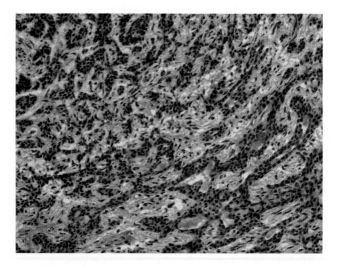

FIG. 4.14 Invasive squamous cell carcinoma.

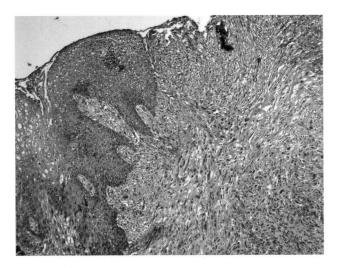

FIG. 4.15 Spindle cell carcinoma in association with squamous cell carcinoma in situ.

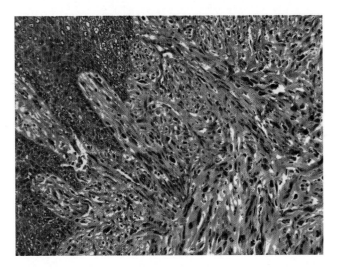

FIG. 4.16 Higher power of Fig. 4.15 showing the intimate relationship between the spindled tumor cells and the dysplastic epithelium.

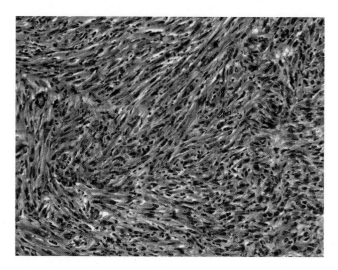

FIG. 4.17 Sarcomatoid change, not to be confused with reactive stromal cells.

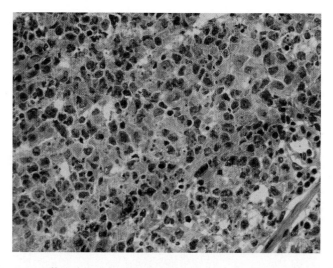

FIG. 4.18 Diffuse large B-cell lymphoma: the tumor cells are discohesive with a high rate of mitosis and apoptosis. Flow cytometry and additional immunostains are highly recommended for final diagnosis of tumors with this morphology. Fresh tissue should be requested at the time of frozen section if an adequate sample for future studies was not provided by the surgeon.

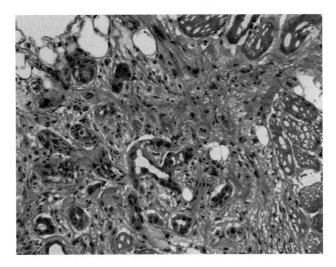

FIG. 4.19 Minor salivary glands with reactive/metaplastic atypia within skeletal muscle of the tongue, not to be confused with invasive carcinoma.

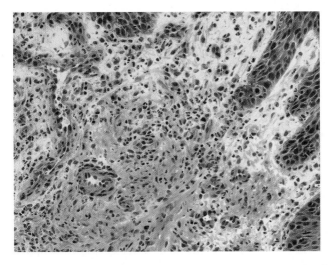

FIG. 4.20 Reactive endothelial cells with vague vessel formation. This finding is the result of prior radiation therapy.

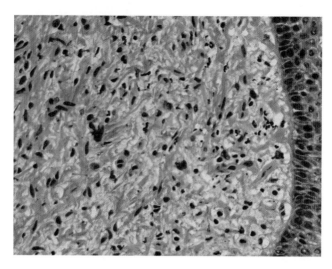

FIG. 4.21 Stromal cells in association with attenuated (thinned) epithelium after radiation therapy.

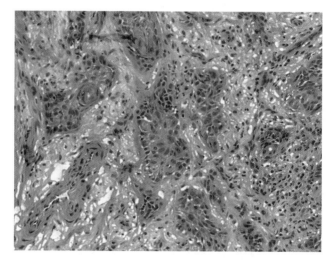

FIG. 4.22 Metaplastic minor salivary glands with a pseudoinvasive pattern, after radiation therapy.

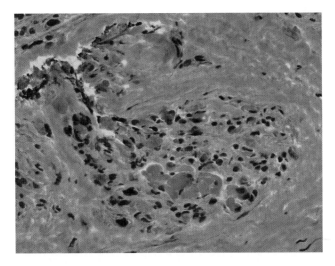

FIG. 4.23 Skeletal muscle with degenerative change after radiation therapy.

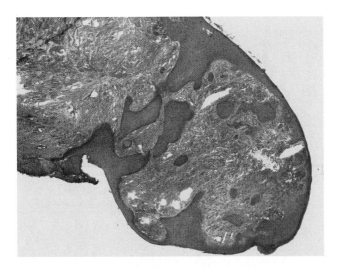

FIG. 4.24 Pseudoepitheliomatous hyperplasia in response to an underlying granular cell tumor from the true vocal cord is a frequent and important diagnostic pitfall. Do not confuse this reactive process with an invasive squamous carcinoma.

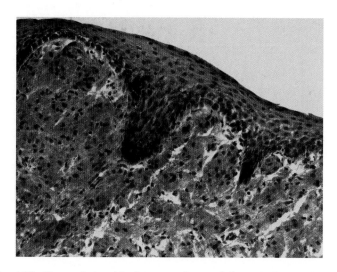

Fig. 4.25 Close relationship between the epithelium and granular cell tumor.

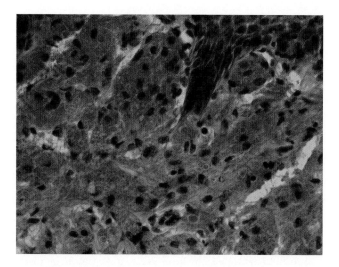

Fig. 4.26 High power showing the typical granular cytoplasm of the granular cell tumor. The nuclei are not enlarged or pleomorphic and no mitoses are observed.

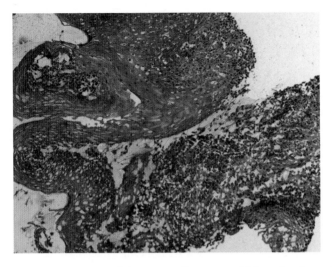

FIG. 4.27 Angiosarcoma of the tongue. Be aware of this entity, do not be confused with reactive vascular endothelium.

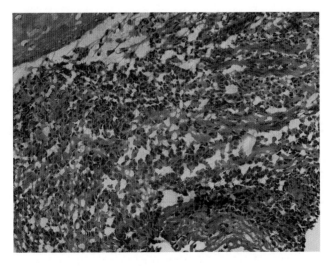

FIG. 4.28 Higher power of Fig. 4.27 demonstrates an anastomosing growth pattern, a typical histologic feature of angiosarcoma.

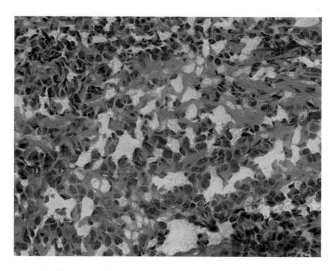

FIG. 4.29   High power of Fig. 4.27 angiosarcoma showing tumor cells with marked atypia, beyond the atypical degree of reactive endothelial cells.

thickness involvement by dysplastic cells. This grading system has been extended to most other organs, including the UADT to some extent, mainly for those lesions without obvious architectural changes (Figs. 4.4, 4.5, 4.11, and 4.12).

Very frequently, squamous dysplasia of the UADT demonstrates obvious architectural disturbance, which is associated with invasive carcinoma (Figs. 4.8–4.10). These histologic features are relatively unique and very important in evaluating the degree of squamous dysplasia.

There are numerous publications on various classifications of squamous dysplasia in the UADT describing the spectrum of histologic changes in relation to their malignant potential. In this chapter, we use the classification and criteria described in WHO Classifications 2005 Pathology and Genetics Head and Neck Tumors.

Hyperplasia. Hyperplasia describes increased cell numbers. This may be in the spinous layer (acanthosis) and/or in the basal/parabasal cell layers (basal cell hyperplasia). The architecture shows regular stratification and there is no cellular atypia. The major change is the increase of cell layers in the upper or the basal part (Figs. 4.2 and 4.3).

Dysplasia. Dysplasia (intraepithelial neoplasia) is used to describe the architectural disturbance accompanied by cytologic atypia. There are four tiers/degrees of squamous dysplasia (1) mild dysplasia, (2) moderate dysplasia, (3) severe dysplasia, and (4) carcinoma in situ:

1. *Mild dysplasia*. Mild dysplasia is defined as architectural disturbance limited to the lower third of the epithelium accompanied by cytologic atypia. Early dysplasia is difficult to reliably diagnose in a consistent manner. The good news is that there is no additional treatment for a diagnosis of mild dysplasia.

2. *Moderate dysplasia*. Architectural disturbance extending into the middle third of the epithelium is the initial criterion for recognizing this category. However, the degree of cytologic atypia may require upgrading. In other words, when the architectural disturbance reaches two thirds of the epithelial thickness and the cytologic atypia is marked, it is appropriate to call it severe dysplasia. In this latter category, full thickness dysplastic involvement is not required for a diagnosis of severe dysplasia. Interestingly, keratinization is very common in these lesions and is associated with the architectural distortion (Figs. 4.6 and 4.7).

   The architectural distortion weighs heavily in assessing the degree of dysplasia and may be more important than the cytologic atypia. This criterion is different from the criterion for uterine cervical dysplasia, which displays less architectural disturbance and less keratinization. This might be a reason that the grading of squamous dysplasia among head and neck pathologists is considered to be of a lower threshold.

   The rational to upgrade is that we often appreciate the invasive component of squamous cell carcinoma directly arising from an area of moderate dysplasia. Unfortunately, there are no reliable histologic features predicting which lesion is going to progress to invasion. Thus, dysplasia in this category should not be ignored and should be treated as if a diagnosis of severe dysplasia has been rendered.

   To my knowledge, there is no scientific explanation for this phenomenon. A personal speculation, which has helped me to remember this phenomenon, is that the keratin may have some locally damaging function, evidenced by two scenarios: first, (a) keratinized odontogenic cyst is a locally aggressive lesion; second a cholesteatoma may extend into the adjacent bone.

3. *Severe dysplasia*. It is defined by the involvement of dysplastic cells and architectural disturbance of greater than two thirds of the epithelial thickness.

4. *Carcinoma in situ*. By definition, malignant transformation has occurred, but invasion is not present in carcinoma in situ. Histologic description is full thickness or almost full thickness architectural abnormalities in the viable cellular layers accompanied by pronounced cytologic atypia (Fig. 4.12 and 4.13). Atypical mitotic figures and abnormal superficial mitoses are commonly seen in carcinoma in situ. Severe dysplasia and carcinoma in situ are separated generally to provide different management guidelines.

Differential Diagnoses

Reactive, regenerative, or reparative squamous epithelium in response to trauma, inflammation, radiation therapy, a tumor, ulceration, or a fungal infection may demonstrate cytologic or architectural disturbances which mimic true dysplasia.

Clinical history is an important piece of information to help avoid overdiagnosis of a malignancy. Morphological identification of the possible etiology of the reactive, regenerative, or reparative change may be identified, such as an underlying tumor (granular cell tumor), fungal infection, inflammation/ulceration or radiation therapy-induced mesenchymal and/or endothelial nuclear enlargement, and hyperchromatism (Figs. 4.19–4.26). The epithelial changes in these cases are generally less pronounced than in dysplasia.

DEFINITION OF A POSITIVE RESECTION MARGIN

It is important to use the same terminology as your clinical colleague when defining a positive resection margin. Pathologically, a positive margin should be defined as a transection of invasive or in situ carcinoma cells. However, the clinical definition of a positive margin implies a risk of recurrence. In our institution, we first report if the tumor is transected (invasive or in situ); if not, then we measure the distance from the tumor cells to the closest margin. The surgeon will make a decision if any additional margin should be obtained considering other parameters. Whether the patient needs any additional therapeutic management, such as chemotherapy and/or radiation therapy, will be decided by the clinician after taking other information into consideration such as tumor staging, extranodal extension, distant metastasis, patient age, and general health condition.

The histologic spectrum illustrated in the accompanying figures and legends can be seen in the process of evaluating the status of resection margins. The tissue will shrink after being removed from the human body. This tissue shrinkage will cause the measurement from the tumor to the margin to be shorter than the clinical distance; such discrepancies should not be surprising.

SIGNIFICANCE OF THE DIFFERENT GRADES OF DYSPLASIA

Dysplasia is a continuum of histologic progression. Although we have well written criteria to grade its severity, the interpretation of the criteria is subjective and this is often compounded by the frozen section artifacts. As a guideline, mild dysplasia will not be treated; moderate dysplasia is within the gray zone; severe dysplasia and carcinoma in situ will be re-excised for a clear margin. These decisions are made depending on the clinical circumstance, such as location of the tumor and potential organ function. Some authors feel that a two-tier system should be used: low grade including mild dysplasia; high grade including moderate and severe dysplasia.

MAJOR DIAGNOSTIC CONSIDERATIONS

- Squamous mucosal precursor lesions – hyperplasia, dysplasia, and squamous cell carcinoma in situ
- Previous therapy – radiation and/or chemotherapy, and/or surgical treatment-induced atypia
- Pseudoepitheliomatous hyperplasia, induced by underlying granular cell tumor or fungal infection (blastomycosis)
- Invasive carcinoma versus reactive stromal cells versus epithelioid endothelial cells
- Squamous papilloma/papillomatosis (no mucocytes and most commonly arising from tongue, tonsil, and uvula)
- Granular cell tumor
- Angiosarcoma
- Lymphoma is not an uncommon disease in the head and neck area. Usually, diffuse large B-cell lymphoma is discohesive and displays obvious malignant histologic features, such as high N/C ratio, tumor necrosis, brisk mitoses, etc. (Fig. 4.18)
- Minor salivary gland tumors do occur in these organs because minor salivary glands exist in the submucosa throughout the aerodigestive tract. Being aware of this possibility is important (for details, refer to Chapter 3)

WHAT SURGEONS NEED TO KNOW INTRAOPERATIVELY TO CHOOSE THE OPTIMAL IMMEDIATE SURGICAL MODALITY

- Establish a correct diagnosis and differentiate it from its benign mimickers to facilitate immediate surgical interventions
- Determine adequacy of resection margins (positive or negative and the distance from the invasive carcinoma)
- Spindle cell carcinoma versus reactive fibrosis
- Assess specimen for the presence or absence of perineural invasion

- Assess the extension of the carcinoma, which may require additional resection
- Determine if sufficient tissue has been obtained or if additional tissue is needed for further studies. For example, a lymphoid proliferation may require additional studies such as immuno-histochemistry and flow cytometry

SPECIMEN HANDLING AND GROSS DIAGNOSIS

Sections from margins can be submitted either *en face* (shaved) or perpendicular to the resection surface. This decision is vital, irre-versible and dependent on the distance from lesion to the resection margin as assessed grossly.

- When margins are macroscopically negative, *en face* sections are sufficient to confirm and document.
- When in doubt, perpendicular sections should be used to verify and measure the microscopic distance to the margin.

Separate submissions of the individual margins by the surgeon might be easier for the pathologist, since the surgeons know where the tissue was obtained. If this is the case, we do not need to spend much time determining where the margins are and how to section them (*en face* or perpendicular); however, we will have to handle a large number of the frozen specimens simultaneously.

USEFUL DIAGNOSTIC PEARLS

Some of the entity-related pearls are described in the figure legends:

- Review of any previous biopsy, surgical, or cytologic specimens may be helpful in correlating with the frozen section to assess reactive changes versus malignancy.
- Communication with the surgeon about the therapy history and finding reactive changes (including endothelial cells, stromal cells, degenerative skeletal muscle, sialometaplasia, acute and chronic inflammation) is useful in evaluating reactive changes versus malignancy.
- Histologic definition of a positive margin is defined by transec-tion of the tumor cells; we can provide the distance from the tumor to the resection margin (tissue shrinks significantly after resection from the human body, especially so for the mucosa).
- When the pathologist has questions about where to sample margins, a close communication with the surgeon regarding a specific area of concern is important.
- The tissue should be mounted on the frozen chuck such that both epithelium and submucosa can be examined; this is

especially important to evaluate if there is invasion, since we heavily rely on the intactness of the basement membrane to determine invasion.

- Drawing a diagram is a practical approach for some specimens without clear anatomic landmarks. When a positive margin is found, we can always use the diagram to explain the findings to the surgeon.

- Depending on the specific scenario, if a margin is at a location that can be resected a few additional millimeters and will not significantly impact the patient's outcome, additional resection might be wise for some atypical cells, which could avoid bringing the patient back for additional surgery or having to put them through radiation therapy.

- As a general rule, when debating benign versus malignant, it is better to err on the benign side, rather than providing a malignant diagnosis resulting in an irreversible radical procedure.

- Depending on the site of the biopsied tissue, a close communication with the clinician is crucial for future management. We may not want to recommend a laryngectomy based on a diagnosis that is not well agreed upon among the pathologists. In this scenario, multiple-site biopsies followed by a close surveillance might be more prudent and may serve the best interests of the patient.

- Discrepancy between frozen section diagnosis and permanent section may be encountered for the margin examined *en face* at frozen section. Orientation is the key to avoiding this type of discrepancy and embedding of the tissue should be carefully handled at the time of frozen section. Intraoperatively, multiple sections with appropriate skips will reduce the incidence of such discrepancy. When this discrepancy occurs, discussion with the surgeon to evaluate the confidence of the frozen section diagnosis is necessary.

- It is not uncommon to find that different levels of the section may show totally different diagnoses. When clinically suspicious, additional levels may reveal the true status of the lesion (margin).

- Spindle cell carcinoma should not be confused with reactive stromal cells. Spindle cell carcinoma is usually associated with an epithelial dysplasia or carcinoma in situ. The spindled tumor cells are diffuse and hypercellular with significant cytologic atypia. Reactive/atypical stromal cells are usually isolated and patchy and not closely associated with epithelial dysplasia. Other accompanying reactive features such as endothelial atypia, inflammation, and/or hyperplastic squamous epithelium are often present (Figs. 4.20–4.22).

- *Useful diagnostic features in architecture and cytology in assessing dysplasia*
  More attention should be given to the overall growth pattern in assessing dysplasia:

  1. Diagnostic clues for the architectural disturbance include the elongation and irregular shapes of the rete pegs, drop-down appearance (giving a pseudoinvasive appearance), irregular epithelial stratification, loss of polarity in the basal cells, abnormal superficial mitoses, premature keratinization in single cells (dyskeratosis), keratin pearls within rete pegs, etc.
  2. The diagnostic features for cytologic dysplasia are no different from the dysplasia criteria in any other organs. Most criteria include the three "S's": the nuclear/cellular size, shape, and space. Significant variations in cellular/nuclear size, shape, and space among these cells are the key features for diagnosing dysplasia. Additional features of dysplasia include increased nuclear–cytoplasmic ratio, atypical mitoses, and prominent nucleoli.

COMMON DIAGNOSTIC PITFALLS

- Some confusions and "lower threshold" for severe dysplasia in head and neck pathology is in part due to the so-called upgrading to severe dysplasia when there is no full thickness of cytologic dysplasia.
- Frozen section artifacts cause an overcall of nondysplastic epithelium to dysplastic.
- Overcalling radiation atypia as invasive carcinoma is a common pitfall.
- Granular cell tumor or fungal infection-induced pseudoepitheliomatous hyperplasia may mimic squamous cell carcinoma (Figs. 4.24–4.26).
- Angiosarcoma of the tongue may be confused with reactive spindle/vascular (granulation) lesion (Figs. 4.27–4.29).
- The organ of Chievitz and odontogenic epithelium are nests of benign epithelium located in the retromolar trigone area. Being aware of their existence could prevent misinterpretation as invasive carcinoma, especially when the tissue is obtained for evaluating a resection margin with a confirmed diagnosis of invasive squamous carcinoma. Rest of Serres, sharing similar histology with the organ of Chievitz is another mimicker simulating a recurrent carcinoma.

- When tissue is obtained from soft tissue or bone of the oral cavity, the possibility of embryonic remnants of dental epithelium should be kept in mind. Rests of Malassez are found in the periodontal ligament near the cementum. Their histology is typically multiple, anastomosing cords, or isolated clusters of round to cuboidal cells with peripheral palisading, commonly about 4–20 in number. They are probably the source of periapical cysts, keratocysts, and other odontogenic tumors.

Chapter 5
Neck

INTRODUCTION

Metastatic tumors to lymph nodes form the main body of neck masses and cystic lesions in the adult patients. The primary malignancies often found in head and neck regions are breast, melanoma, lung, thyroid, or occult metastatic squamous cell carcinoma. That being said, benign primary neck lesions such as branchial cleft cyst, thyroglossal duct, etc., should be carefully differentiated from metastatic tumors. An overtreatment such as neck lymph node dissections, could result if these benign entities are misdiagnosed as a metastatic cystic squamous carcinoma.

In children, the majority of the neck masses and cystic lesions are benign in nature, most commonly developmental anomalies, followed by inflammatory response, and in rare cases malignant tumors.

MAJOR DIAGNOSTIC CONSIDERATIONS
- Cystic lesions include cystic metastatic squamous carcinoma to cervical lymph nodes, branchial cleft cysts, thyroglossal duct cysts, cystic hygromas (lymphangiomas), teratomas, dermoid cysts, and thymic cysts.
- Lymphomas include Hodgkin's and non-Hodgkin's lymphoma.
- Paraganglioma (carotid body tumor) can be seen throughout the body; its most frequent representation in the head and neck area is carotid body tumor at the bifurcation of the internal and external carotid arteries. The location of the tumor is an important hint for this entity (Figs. 5.1 and 5.2).
- Schwannoma located in the internal auditory canal is also called *acoustic neuroma*. Schwannoma can also be seen in any branch of the cervical nerves (Fig. 5.3).

Q.J. Zhai, *Frozen Section Library: Head and Neck*, Frozen Section Library 5, DOI 10.1007/978-0-387-95988-7_5, © Springer Science+Business Media, LLC 2011

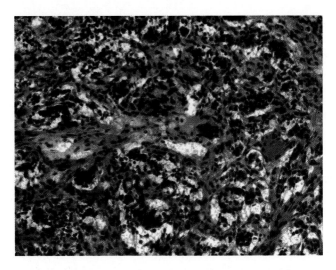

FIG. 5.1 Paraganglioma: small nests of uniform tumor cells in a rich vascular stroma.

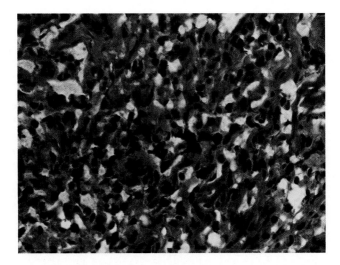

FIG. 5.2 High power of a paraganglioma displays irregular, large, hyperchromatic nuclei (neuroendocrine atypia), a typical feature of this lesion.

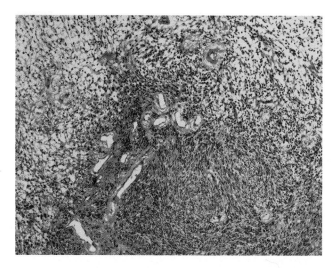

FIG. 5.3   Schwannoma at low power shows an alterative pattern, hypercellular and hypocellular areas, and palisading arrays of nuclei (Verocay bodies).

- Reactive changes within a cervical lymph node can generate a false-positive diagnosis (Figs. 5.4 and 5.5).
- Sarcoidosis may be observed within a cervical lymph node (Fig. 5.6).
- Metastatic thyroid carcinoma to neck lymph nodes or soft tissue may be an unexpected finding without a known history of thyroid cancer (Figs. 5.7 and 5.8).
- Metastatic squamous cell carcinoma to neck soft tissue may be an unexpected finding when there is no known history of a primary squamous cell carcinoma (Fig. 5.9).

WHAT SURGEONS NEED TO KNOW INTRAOPERATIVELY TO CHOOSE THE OPTIMAL IMMEDIATE SURGICAL MODALITY

- Determining the nature of the lesions (metastatic carcinoma, primary malignancy including lymphoma or congenital cysts) to plan/evaluate the extent of the surgery
- Evaluating lymph nodes to determine a metastatic or a primary disease. For a metastatic carcinoma, they may start obtaining biopsies from different sites, looking for the origin. If it is a lymphoid process, they need to know if the tissue is representative and sufficient for an additional hematopathology workup
- Determining if the margins are clear for a resection of a known tumor

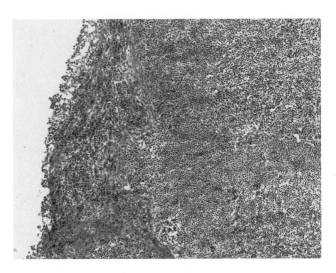

FIG. 5.4 Plasmacytosis (false-positive) node: there is a space-occupying focus at the periphery (capsule) of the node. A metastatic tumor needs to be ruled out.

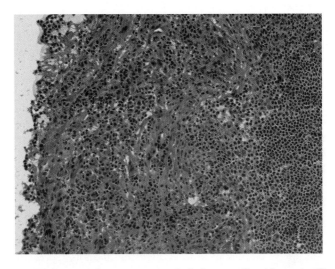

FIG. 5.5 High power demonstrates typical plasma cells without significant atypia in the worrisome focus in Fig. 5.4. Subsequent immunostains confirmed a reactive process.

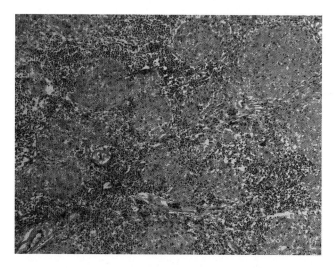

FIG. 5.6 Sarcoidosis in a cervical lymph node: non-necrotizing confluent granulomata, highly suggestive of sarcoidosis. Additional tissue should be requested for culture, if available; and special stains (GMS and AFB) should be performed.

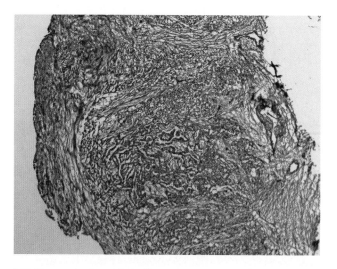

FIG. 5.7 Metastatic thyroid papillary carcinoma to soft tissue in the neck with no previous known history of thyroid carcinoma.

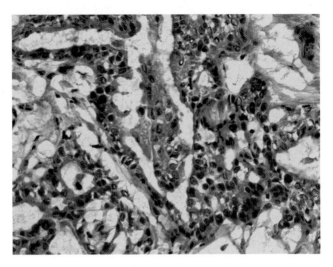

FIG. 5.8 Higher power of the previous case shows typical cytology of thyroid papillary carcinoma.

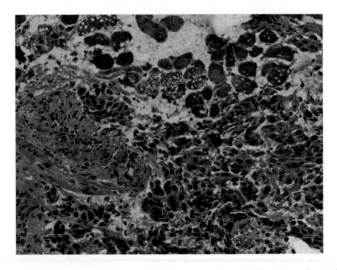

FIG. 5.9 Metastatic squamous cell carcinoma to the skeletal muscle in the neck, with no known primary.

- Any perineural invasion, so the surgeon can decide to sacrifice a particular nerve branch. A conservative approach is to limit the procedure and wait for the final result from permanent sections

SPECIMEN HANDLING AND GROSS DIAGNOSIS

- Gross appearance of a branchial cleft cyst is usually unilocular with a central cavity. The cyst is lined by relatively thin and smooth inner wall. Solid areas can occasionally be seen due to inflammatory and reactive response to rupture of the cyst.
- Orientation with the help of the surgeon is critical before the specimen is cut.
- A smear or touch preparation can be useful, especially for small biopsy material.
- For a lymph node, it is always a good idea to find out the clinical indications before submitting the whole tissue to frozen section.
- Neck dissection for nodal metastasis is a frequent specimen we encounter. Division of specimen into different levels by the surgeon should be encouraged for intraoperative consultation or permanent examination, since they know the details of the regional anatomy and procedure.

USEFUL DIAGNOSTIC PEARLS

Histologic Features of Cystic Squamous Cell Carcinoma to the Neck Lymph Nodes

If there is a history of primary squamous cell carcinoma, it would be a good practice to compare the primary tumor with the metastatic disease. However, if there is no known history, histologic evaluation of the cystic lymphoepithelial lesions would be a last resort to diagnose a metastatic squamous cell carcinoma. Cases with obvious carcinoma features including loss of polarity, frequent mitoses, and cellular anaplasia, would not be difficult to diagnose a metastatic squamous cell carcinoma (Figs. 5.10 and 5.11). Diagnosing cases of "low-grade" metastatic carcinoma at frozen section is challenging.

The majority of occult metastatic squamous cell carcinomas arise from the tonsillar area, and they usually show the following morphologic features (Fig. 5.12):

1. Large unilocular cyst with a thick fibrous capsule formation (occasionally multiple small cysts can be seen as well), predominately a cystic lesion with only focal areas of solid growth
2. Cystic spaces lined by a squamous or transitional epithelium arranged in strips of epithelium of relatively uniform thickness, with areas maintaining the surface maturation
3. No prominent degree of anaplasia; the cells recapitulate the normal tonsillar crypt epithelium

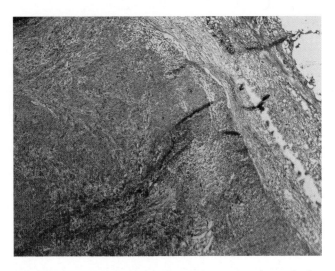

FIG. 5.10 Solid sheets of squamous cell carcinoma at the subcapsular location with adjacent residual lymphoid tissue. This histology is most consistent with a known primary squamous cell carcinoma.

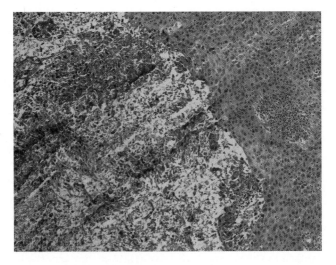

FIG. 5.11 Central necrosis, tissue debris, and keratinization are often seen in a lymph node positive for metastatic squamous cell carcinoma.

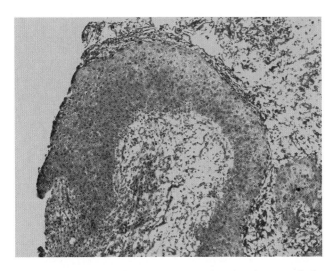

FIG. 5.12 Metastatic squamous carcinoma with cystic changes. The linings of the cystic structures are of a transitional cell look without keratinization, recapitulating the tonsillar epithelium. The tumor cells are relatively bland and no anaplasia is present. This is a common finding for a cystic metastatic squamous carcinoma with no known primary site at the time of frozen section diagnosis. A significant proportion of these cases are found to have a tonsillar primary after extensive searching.

4. With careful searching and necessary sectioning, atypia beyond a reactive change encountered in benign bronchial cysts will be found.

Common Histologic Features of Benign Cervical Cysts

1. The lining of a branchial cleft cyst is mostly composed of a simple keratinizing squamous epithelium. The occasional presence of ciliated pseudostratified respiratory epithelium can be a helpful histologic finding favoring a benign diagnosis. Atypia from a reactive response is a diagnostic pitfall to keep in mind (Figs. 5.13–5.15).
2. Thyroglossal duct often contains a portion of benign thyroid tissue. Benign keratinizing squamous lining can be seen as well. The central location differentiates it from the metastatic lymph node.
3. Hassall's corpuscles are found in thymic cysts.
4. Lymphangioma is lined by benign lymphatic endothelial cells.
5. Frozen sections are commonly requested for these benign cysts. The most important differential diagnosis is metastatic squamous cell carcinoma with cystic change.

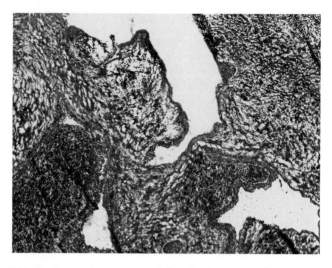

Fig. 5.13   Benign cystic structure with lymphoid aggregates identified within a branchial cleft cyst. There is no significant cellular atypia.

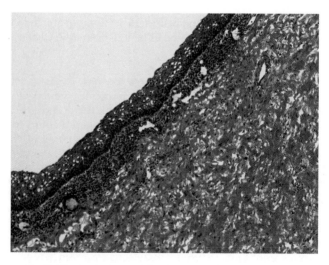

Fig. 5.14   The lining of a branchial cleft cyst is a simple keratinizing squamous epithelium with epithelial maturation.

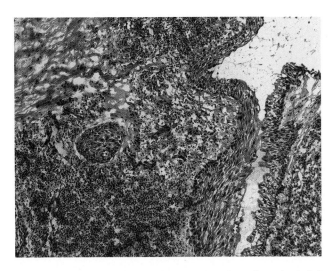

FIG. 5.15 Reactive atypia and pseudoinvasion within a branchial cleft cyst should not be confused with a metastatic squamous cell carcinoma.

- When markedly sclerosing fibrous bands are seen, the possibility of sclerosing nodular Hodgkin's lymphoma should be ruled out before calling it reactive. A touch preparation can be useful to show the mixed cellularity and Reed–Sternberg cells (Figs. 5.16–5.18).
- Determination of specimen adequacy for special tests, such as cultures for a possible infectious process (granulomatous inflammation) (Fig. 5.19), personalized therapy protocol (molecular studies), or flow cytometry.
- Diagnostic (sufficient) fresh tissue is obtained from a lymphoproliferative process, so that additional studies such as immunohistochemistry, flow cytometry, cytogenetic, and molecular tests can be performed at a later time. If not comfortable that sufficient tissue has already been provided for these studies, additional tissue should be requested immediately. By doing this, we can avoid another surgical procedure to obtain the diagnostic tissue. If no immediate therapy will be implemented at the time of frozen section, saving the valuable tissue for a thorough investigation later is the best option at the time of the intraoperative consultation (Figs. 5.20 and 5.21).

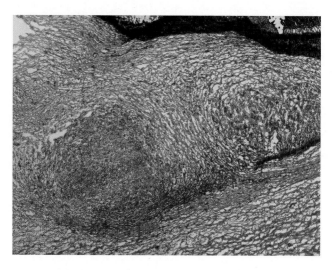

FIG. 5.16 Hodgkin's lymphoma. Nodular and sclerosing pattern should remind us of a Hodgkin's lymphoma.

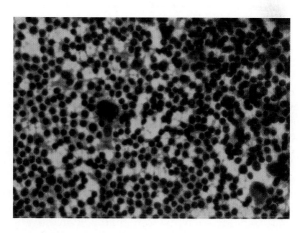

FIG. 5.17 Touch preparation of the above case shows typical Reed–Sternberg cells.

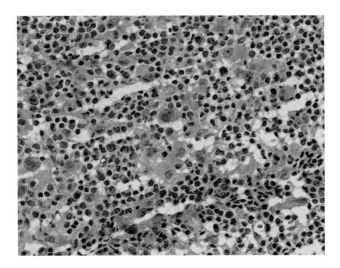

FIG. 5.18 Frozen section of the above case shows typical Reed–Sternberg cells.

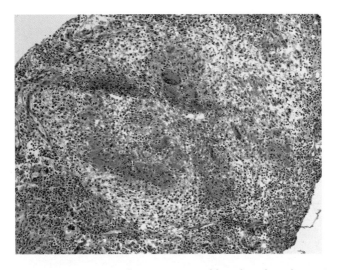

FIG. 5.19 Necrotizing granuloma in a cervical lymph node: a diagnosis of "negative for malignancy" can be made. Additional tissue for microbiology culture should be requested; and special stains (GMS and AFB) will be performed on the permanent sections.

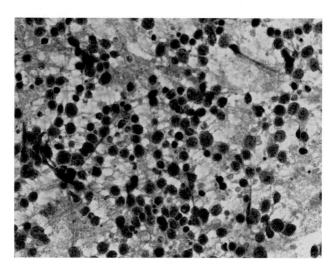

Fɪɢ. 5.20 Diffuse large B-cell lymphoma. Touch preparation shows a diffuse process; the cells are large (compared to the lymphocytes) and are not cohesive.

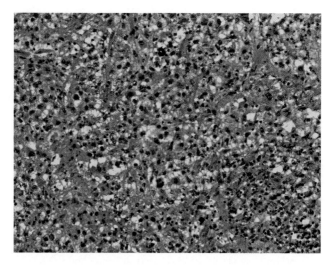

Fɪɢ. 5.21 Frozen section of the above case demonstrates discohesive tumor cells with necrosis and mitoses. Additional fresh tissue should be requested for additional tests.

COMMON DIAGNOSTIC PITFALLS

- A benign cyst with reactive atypia may be misdiagnosed as a well-differentiated metastatic squamous cell carcinoma.
- Reactive changes within a lymph node may generate a false-positive diagnosis and subsequently lead to numerous biopsies searching for primary neoplasm and/or a neck dissection.
- Thick fibrous bands within a sclerosing nodular Hodgkin's lymphoma may be misinterpreted as a reactive process.
- It is better to defer a lymphoproliferative process to additional lymphoma workup, rather than struggle to reach an accurate diagnosis at the time of intraoperative consultation.

Chapter 6
Head and Neck Presentations of Intracranial Lesions

Ady Kendler and Qihui "Jim" Zhai

INTRODUCTION

Because of the close proximity of the intracranial compartment to head and neck sites, central nervous system (CNS) lesions may be encountered in this region, as primary tumors, developmental or traumatic displacements, and due to direct extension from the brain or meninges. Awareness of CNS lesions (many of which are more easily identified on intraoperative touch/smear preparations made from the typically scant tissue provided) will avoid misdiagnosis during surgery and on permanent specimens. Clinical and radiologic information, of course, is very helpful. The histology of these entities, described below, is identical to their intracranial counterpart.

MAJOR DIAGNOSTIC CONSIDERATIONS
- Meningioma
- CNS tissue (heterotopia)
- Pituitary adenoma

WHAT SURGEONS NEED TO KNOW INTRAOPERATIVELY TO CHOOSE THE OPTIMAL IMMEDIATE SURGICAL MODALITY
- They need to know the diagnosis (or at least the differential diagnosis) of the lesion, and if it is benign or malignant (e.g., meningioma vs. carcinoma or pituitary adenoma vs. small cell carcinoma).

A. Kendler and Q.J. Zhai
Department of Pathology and Laboratory Medicine, University of Cincinnati, 234 Goodman St., Cincinnati, OH 45219, USA

Q.J. Zhai, *Frozen Section Library: Head and Neck*, Frozen Section Library 5, DOI 10.1007/978-0-387-95988-7_6, © Springer Science+Business Media, LLC 2011

- In the case of a biopsy, "adequate/diagnostic" or "neoplastic tissue" may be sufficient for intraoperative diagnosis.
- Margins may be submitted for evaluation.
- The potential behavior of the lesion is important. If the lesion is due to direct extension (e.g., meningioma) versus a primary or a metastasis, the surgeon may want to corroborate the clinical impression.

SPECIMEN HANDLING AND GROSS DIAGNOSIS

In the case of small tissue biopsies for diagnosis, an attempt should be made to save some pieces for permanent sections as well as smears/frozen sections. Margins should, of course, be frozen or smeared in their entirety. As discussed below, intraoperative smear diagnosis may be helpful, either as an adjunct to frozen section or replacing it. A judgment as to whether a smear preparation will be useful (e.g., a firm fibrous or boney specimen will not smear well) should be made.

USEFUL DIAGNOSTIC PEARLS
Extracranial Meningioma

- Intraoperative smear (between two glass slides, with immediate fixation in alcohol) shows the typical meningothelial cells, with round or oval speckled "neuroendocrine" nuclei, very low N/C ratio, and a syncytial pattern (i.e., cell borders are not seen, rather multiple nuclei lie within a "syncytium" of cytoplasm). Whorls may be few or abundant, as are nuclear pseudoinclusions (see Fig. 6.1).
- Smear preparation will show the typical whorls and syncytial pattern in meningioma (Fig. 6.1), and will distinguish meningioma from the discohesive, "hepatoid" and physaliferous cells of chordoma (see Figs. 6.2–6.4 for smear and H&Es of chordoma). Even immunostains on permanents may not be helpful (i.e., both may stain for S100 and EMA/keratins).
- Meningiomas may present in the temporal bone, paranasal sinuses, or nasopharynx/lateral pharyngeal wall, either due to direct extension from the meninges or from growth from ectopic intratemporal meningothelial rests. Approximately, 6% of all meningiomas arise from the anterior or posterior surface of the temporal bone; 70% of these have both intracranial and intratemporal components. The 2007 WHO classification has seven well-defined benign (WHO grade 1) variants of meningioma (meningothelial, fibrous, transitional, psammomatous, angiomatous, microcystic, and secretory), two benign subtypes with variable features (lymphoplasmacyte-rich and metaplastic),

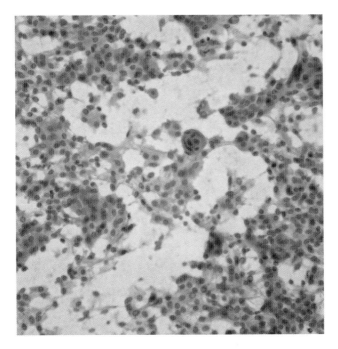

FIG. 6.1 Meningioma: smear preparation shows typical syncytial appearance, low nucleus/cytoplasm ratio, whorls, and nuclear pseudoinclusions.

three atypical subtypes (atypical, clear cell, and chordoid; WHO grade 2) – which tend to recur and may be treated with radiotherapy, and three malignant types (malignant NOS, papillary and rhabdoid; WHO grade 3). Because of the different histologic patterns of meningioma, the differential diagnosis may include carcinoma, spindled cell tumors including soft tissue tumors such as hemangiopericytoma/solitary fibrous tumor and synovial sarcoma, salivary gland tumors such as myoepithelioma, and middle ear tumors such as paraganglioma.

Extracranial Brain Tissue
- Nasal heterotopia (nasal "glioma") is a congenital displacement, or "encephalocele" of CNS tissue in the nasal region.
- This lesion is thought to be due to failure of retraction of the developing frontal lobe through the foramen cecum (reviewed in AFIP fascicle #26, 3rd series, p. 119), resulting in trapped brain tissue within the posterior nasal cavity (25%), subcutaneous anterior nasal tissue, or a combination of both.

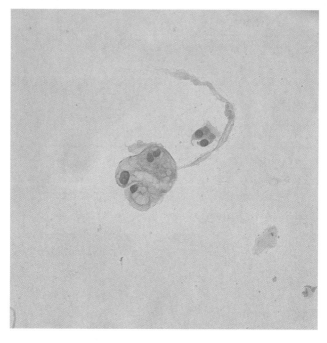

FIG. 6.2   Chordoma: smear preparation highlights physaliferous cells.

- Rarely, CNS heterotopia has been described in the nasopharynx, palate, tonsillar, and pterygoid fossa.
- A frozen section can create artifacts which may make CNS tissue difficult to visualize. These are more easily seen on a smear preparation, which highlights neuroglial tissue in dramatic fashion (see Fig. 6.5 for smear preparation and Figs. 6.6–6.8 for histology).
- Smear preparation can also reveal CNS tissue in acquired encephaloceles, for example, temporal lobe herniation into the middle ear which may occur in patients after trauma, postsurgery, or inflammation.

Pituitary Adenoma
- A touch preparation or smear preparation, if the tissue is not entirely fibrotic, may reveal the monotonous, bland neuroendocrine cells with abundant cytoplasm typical of pituitary adenoma, ruling out entities such as carcinoma, melanoma, lymphoma, meningioma and solitary fibrous tumor/hemangiopericytoma, except possibly paraganglioma, which may be morphologically similar (see Fig. 6.9).

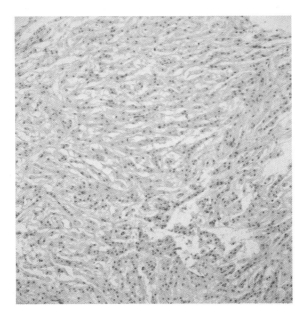

FIG. 6.3 Chordoma: frozen section shows myxoid matrix and cords or groups of "hepatoid cells," a pattern that can be seen in frozen sections of chordoid meningioma.

COMMON DIAGNOSTIC PITFALLS

- Extracranial MeningiomaFrozen section (see Fig. 6.10) may show an infiltrating epithelioid, spindled, or even chordoid neoplasm (differential can include carcinoma, soft tissue tumor, chordoma, or melanoma). Classic features of meningioma (psammoma bodies, lobules, and whorls) may be absent or difficult to visualize on frozen section, but may be more easily seen on smear preparation (Fig. 6.1 and see the section "Useful Diagnostic Pearls").

- An uncommon variant of meningioma is the chordoid meningioma; this is a rare variant, corresponding to a WHO grade 2 (atypical) meningioma which, though benign, is more aggressive than WHO grade 1 meningiomas (recurrence risk is approximately 60% for grade 2 vs. 20% for grade 1 tumors), and these may be treated with radiation. Chordoid meningioma can be easily confused with chordoma on frozen section (mucoid background with clusters of epithelioid cells; see the section "Useful Diagnostic Pearls" and Figs. 6.2–6.4 and 6.11), especially in the case of an invasive clival/sphenoid sinus mass.

- Meningiomas may present as an invasive, epithelioid neoplasm in the temporal bone, paranasal sinuses, or nasopharynx/lateral

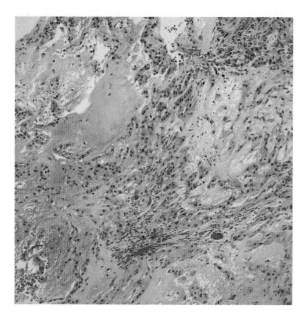

FIG. 6.4   Chordoma: H&E (even the permanent) may be difficult to distinguish from chordoid meningioma.

pharyngeal wall. Differential diagnosis includes a carcinoma and may be difficult on frozen section.

Extracranial Brain Tissue
• Nasal heterotopia (nasal "glioma") is a congenital displacement, or "encephalocele" of CNS tissue in the nasal region. A frozen section can create artifacts which may make CNS tissue difficult to visualize, even if one thinks of this possibility and searches for neurons and glia. Smear preparation may be diagnostic.

Pituitary Adenoma
• Benign pituitary adenomas may be very invasive and may present as sphenoid sinus or clival lesions due to direct invasion from the sella turcica. Rarely, ectopic rests of pituitary tissue in these locations may develop into an adenoma.
• Frozen sections of tissue from these areas usually show fibrous tissue with crushed nests of "small blue" cells; thus, the differential is broad and includes primary sinus neoplasms (e.g., sinonasal undifferentiated carcinoma, small cell carcinoma, squamous carcinoma, carcinoid tumor, lymphoma, plasmacytoma, meningioma, paraganglioma, chordoma, and melanoma).

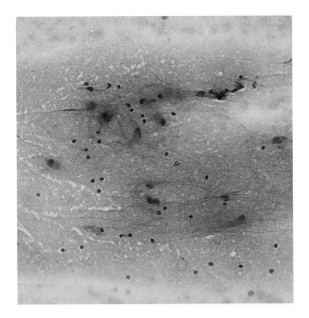

FIG. 6.5 CNS heterotopia: smear preparation shows a neuroglial background and reactive astrocytes, confirming CNS tissue.

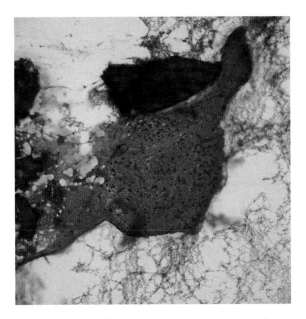

FIG. 6.6 CNS heterotopia: frozen section – brain tissue on a frozen section may be difficult to identify.

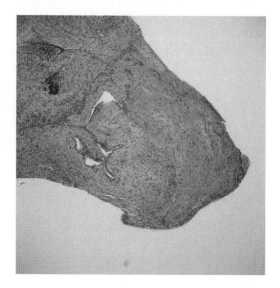

Fig. 6.7 CNS heterotopia: permanent sections may show CNS tissue with gliosis (even this may be challenging to distinguish from fibrous stroma).

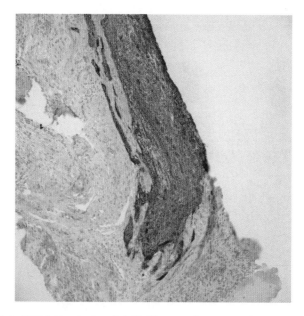

Fig. 6.8 CNS heterotopia: glial fibrillary acidic protein (GFAP) immunohistochemistry highlights CNS tissue.

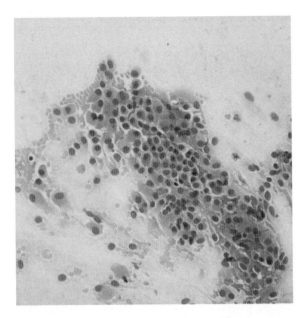

FIG. 6.9 Pituitary adenoma: touch preparation confirms bland neuroendo-crine cells and can rule out entities in the differential diagnosis (see text).

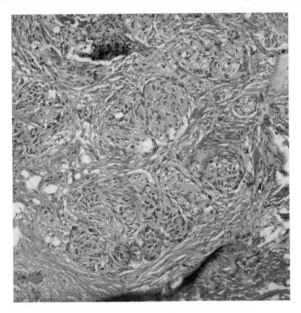

FIG. 6.10 Meningioma: frozen section may not show psammoma bodies or whorls and may show infiltration of fibroadipose tissue (a benign feature of meningioma), which could be mistaken for infiltrating carcinoma.

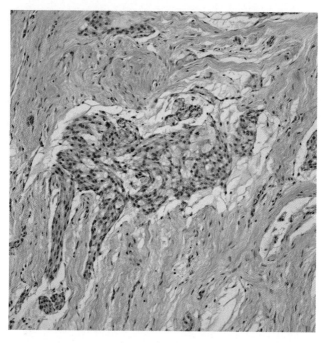

Fɪɢ. 6.11 Chordoid meningioma: H&E (frozen or permanent) may be difficult to distinguish from chordoma.

Suggested Readings

Acurio A, Taxy J. Head and neck. In: *Biopsy Interpretation: The Frozen Section*. Taxy J Husain A, Montag A, editors, pp. 149–171. Lippincott Williams & Wilkins, Philadelphia, PA, 2009

Badoual C, Rousseau A, Heudes D, Carnot F, Danel C, Meatchi T, Hans1 S, Bruneval P, Brasnu1 D, Laccourreye O. Evaluation of frozen section diagnosis in 721 parotid gland lesions. *Histopathology* 2006; 49, 538–558

Ellis GL, Auclair PL. *Atlas of Tumor Pathology*. Tumors of the Salivary Glands, Third Series, Vol. 17. Armed Forces Institute of Pathology Press, Washington, DC, 1996

Fu YS, Wenig BM, Abemayor E, Wenig BL. *Head and Neck Pathology with Clinical Correlations*. Churchill Livingstone, Philadelphia, PA, 2001

Gale N, Pilch BZ, Sidransky D, Westra WH, Califano J. Epithelial precursor lesions. In: *Pathology & Genetics Head and Neck Tumors WHO Classification*. Barnes L, Eveson J, Reichart P, Sidransky D, editors, pp. 140–143. IARC, Lyon, 2005

Gnepp D. *Diagnostic Surgical Pathology of the Head and Neck*, 2nd ed. Saunders/Elsevier, Philadelphia, PA, 2009

Heller K, Attie JN, Dubner S. Accuracy of frozen section in the evaluation of salivary tumors. *The American Journal of Surgery* 1993; 166, 424–427

Mills SE, Gaffey M, Frierson HF. *Atlas of Tumor Pathology*. Tumors of the Upper Aerodigestive Tract and Ear, Third Series, Vol. 26. Armed Forces Institute of Pathology Press, Washington, DC, 2000

Neville BW, Damm DD, Allen CM, Bouquot JE. *Oral and Maxillofacial Pathology*. 3rd ed. Saunders/Elsevier, Philadelphia, PA, 2009

Seethala RR, LiVolsi VA, Baloch ZW. Relative accuracy of fine-needle aspiration and frozen section in the diagnosis of lesions of the parotid gland. *Head & Neck* 2005; 27, 217–223

Thompson LDR. *Head and Neck Pathology*. Churchill Livingstone/Elsevier, Philadelphia, PA, 2006

Thompson LDR, Heffner DK. The clinical importance of cystic squamous cell carcinomas in the neck: a study of 136 cases. *Cancer* 1998; 82, 944–956

Wenig BM. *Atlas of Head and Neck Pathology*, 2nd ed. Saunders/Elsevier, Philadelphia, PA, 2008

Wong DSY. Frozen section during parotid surgery revisited: efficacy of its applications and changing trend of indications. *Head & Neck* 2002; 24, 191–197

Zbären P, Nuyens M, Loosli H, Stauffer E. Diagnostic accuracy of fine-needle aspiration cytology and frozen section in primary parotid carcinoma. *Cancer* 2004; 100, 1876–1883

Zbären P, Guélat D, Loosli H, Stauffer E. Parotid tumors: fine-needle aspiration and/or frozen section. *Otolaryngology – Head and Neck Surgery* 2008; 139, 811–815

Zheng JW, Song XY, Nie XG. The accuracy of clinical examination versus frozen section in the diagnosis of parotid masses. *Journal of Maxillofacial Surgery* 1997; 55, 29–31

Index

Q.J. Zhai, *Frozen Section Library: Head and Neck*, Frozen Section Library 5,
DOI 10.1007/978-0-387-95988-7, © Springer Science+Business Media, LLC 2011

Printed in the United States of America